BRIGHAM AND WOMEN'S
EXPERTS' APPROACH TO
RHEUMATOLOGY

Jonathan S. Coblyn, MD
Director of Clinical Rheumatology
Director for the Center for Arthritis and Joint Diseases
Vice Chairman-Department of Medicine
Brigham and Women's Hospital
Associate Professor of Medicine
Harvard Medical School

Bonnie Bermas, MD
Clinical Director of the Lupus Center
Division of Allergy, Immunology, and Rheumatology
Brigham and Women's Hospital
Harvard Medical School

Michael Weinblatt, MD
Co-Director of Clinical Rheumatology
Associate Director for the Center for Arthritis and Joint Diseases
Brigham and Women's Hospital
Professor of Medicine
Harvard Medical School

Simon Helfgott, MD
Director of Education and Fellowship Training
Division of Allergy, Immunology, and Rheumatology
Brigham and Women's Hospital
Harvard Medical School

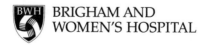

BRIGHAM AND
WOMEN'S HOSPITAL

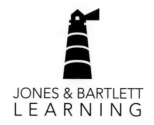

JONES & BARTLETT
LEARNING

D1205743

World Headquarters
Jones & Bartlett Learning
40 Tall Pine Drive
Sudbury, MA 01776
978-443-5000
info@jblearning.com
www.jblearning.com

Jones & Bartlett Learning
Canada
6339 Ormindale Way
Mississauga, Ontario L5V 1J2
Canada

Jones & Bartlett Learning
International
Barb House, Barb Mews
London W6 7PA
United Kingdom

Jones & Bartlett Learning books and products are available through most bookstores and online booksellers. To contact Jones & Bartlett Learning directly, call 800-832-0034, fax 978-443-8000, or visit our website, www.jblearning.com.

Substantial discounts on bulk quantities of Jones & Bartlett Learning publications are available to corporations, professional associations, and other qualified organizations. For details and specific discount information, contact the special sales department at Jones & Bartlett Learning via the above contact information or send an email to specialsales@jblearning.com.

The authors, editor, and publisher have made every effort to provide accurate information. However, they are not responsible for errors, omissions, or for any outcomes related to the use of the contents of this book and take no responsibility for the use of the products and procedures described. Treatments and side effects described in this book may not be applicable to all people; likewise, some people may require a dose or experience a side effect that is not described herein. Drugs and medical devices are discussed that may have limited availability controlled by the Food and Drug Administration (FDA) for use only in a research study or clinical trial. Research, clinical practice, and government regulations often change the accepted standard in this field. When consideration is being given to use of any drug in the clinical setting, the healthcare provider or reader is responsible for determining FDA status of the drug, reading the package insert, and reviewing prescribing information for the most up-to-date recommendations on dose, precautions, and contraindications, and determining the appropriate usage for the product. This is especially important in the case of drugs that are new or seldom used.

Production Credits
Senior Acquisitions Editor: Alison Hankey
Editorial Assistant: Sara Cameron
Production Director: Amy Rose
Associate Production Editor: Jessica deMartin
Associate Marketing Manager: Marion Kerr
V.P., Manufacturing and Inventory Control: Therese Connell
Composition: Nicolazzo Productions
Printing and Binding: Malloy, Inc.

Cover Credits
Cover Design: Scott Moden
Cover Image: Courtesy of Dr. Michael Weinblatt
Cover Printing: Malloy, Inc.

Library of Congress Cataloging-in-Publication Data

Brigham and Women's experts' approach to rheumatology / [edited by] Jonathan S. Coblyn ... [et al.].
    p. ; cm.
Other title: Experts' approach to rheumatology
Includes bibliographical references and index.
ISBN-13: 978-0-7637-6916-1
ISBN-10: 0-7637-6916-9
1. Rheumatology—Handbooks, manuals, etc. I. Coblyn, Jonathan S. II. Brigham and Women's Hospital. III. Title: Experts' approach to rheumatology.
[DNLM: 1. Rheumatic Diseases—diagnosis. 2. Rheumatic Diseases--therapy. WE 544 B855 2011]
RC927.B685 2011
616.7'23—dc22
                                2010000303

6048
Printed in the United States of America
14 13 12 11 10   10 9 8 7 6 5 4 3 2 1

DEDICATION

This book is dedicated to our mentor, Ronald J. Anderson, MD, who has been on the faculties of Harvard Medical School and the Brigham and Women's Hospital since the early 1970s. For close to four decades, Dr. Anderson has taught countless medical students, residents, and fellows about the field of rheumatology and, more importantly, life. His intelligence, compassion, kindness, thoughtfulness, and sense of humor have helped us to become better physicians and human beings.

In addition, we are fortunate to interact with a wonderful group of trainees who constantly amaze us with their intelligence, hard work, and passion for rheumatology. Finally, we would like to thank our patients who, on a daily basis, teach us something new about medicine.

CONTENTS

EDITORS AND CONTRIBUTORS

EDITORS

Jonathan S. Coblyn, MD
Director of Clinical Rheumatology
Director for the Center for Arthritis and
  Joint Diseases
Vice-Chairman, Department of Medicine
Brigham and Women's Hospital
Harvard Medical School

Bonnie Bermas, MD
Clinical Director of the Lupus Center
Division of Allergy, Immunology, and
  Rheumatology
Brigham and Women's Hospital
Harvard Medical School

ASSOCIATE EDITORS

Michael Weinblatt, MD
Co-Director of Clinical Rheumatology
Associate Director for the Center for
  Arthritis and Joint Diseases
Brigham and Women's Hospital
Professor of Medicine
Harvard Medical School

Simon Helfgott, MD
Director of Education and Fellowship
  Training
Division of Allergy, Immunology, and
  Rheumatology
Brigham and Women's Hospital
Harvard Medical School

CONTRIBUTORS

Alan G. Cole, MD
Division of Endocrinology, Diabetes,
  and Hypertension
Brigham and Women's Hospital
Harvard Medical School

Joerg Ermann, MD
Rheumatology Fellow
Division of Rheumatology
Brigham and Women's Hospital
Harvard Medical School

Sonali Desai, MD
Instructor in Medicine
Harvard Medical School
Division of Rheumatology
Brigham and Women's Hospital

Roger Han, MD
Department of Radiology
Brigham and Women's Hospital

Rumey Ishizawar, MD
Rheumatology Fellow
Division of Rheumatology
Brigham and Women's Hospital
Harvard Medical School

Martin A. Kriegel, MD, PhD
Clinical Fellow in Rheumatology
Harvard Medical School
Division of Rheumatology
Brigham and Women's Hospital

Yvonne C. Lee, MD
Instructor in Medicine
Harvard Medical School
Division of Rheumatology, Immunology
     and Allergy
Brigham and Women's Hospital

Katherine P. Liao, MD
Rheumatology Fellow
Division of Rheumatology
Brigham and Women's Hospital
Harvard Medical School

Thorvardur Jon Love, MD
Rheumatology Fellow
Division of Rheumatology
Brigham and Women's Hospital
Harvard Medical School

Soumya Raychaudhuri, MD, PhD
Rheumatology Fellow
Division of Rheumatology
Brigham and Women's Hospital
Harvard Medical School

Susan Y. Ritter, MD, PhD
Rheumatology Fellow
Division of Rheumatology
Brigham and Women's Hospital
Harvard Medical School

Kichul Shin, MD, PhD
Rheumatology Fellow
Division of Rheumatology
Brigham and Women's Hospital
Harvard Medical School

Derrick J. Todd, MD, PhD
Instructor in Medicine
Harvard Medical School
Division of Rheumatology
Brigham and Women's Hospital

PREFACE

I am sure you are asking yourself—why would anyone publish a medical textbook about rheumatology in this era of multiple publications and easy Internet access? That, in fact, may be part of the problem. There may be too much information for a primary care practitioner to assimilate in a timely way to address a patient's problem when he or she is in your office. Many publications are burdensome, and the Internet, although timely, can be challenging to access during a busy day.

Moreover, we would argue that although rheumatologic symptoms are amongst the most common reasons patients present to their primary care provider, rheumatology is one of the most poorly taught disciplines in medical schools; is often misunderstood by healthcare providers; and has a myriad of laboratory tests, features, and clinical syndromes that are confusing. It is for this reason that we have written this book. It attempts to summarize and simplify the important aspects of rheumatology and to help sort out among the various symptoms, signs, and laboratory tests that distinguish rheumatologic disorders. We hope to provide you with an understandable and reasonable treatment plan for these disorders. This text hopefully will be a source for easily discovered information regarding this discipline—useful information that can be obtained quickly to help contribute to the care of the patient.

CHAPTER 1

Approach to the Patient with Musculoskeletal Disease

Soumya Raychaudhuri, MD, PhD

OVERVIEW

Rheumatic disease encompasses a wide range of diseases and illnesses that are character-ized by their propensity to affect the bones, joints, and soft tissues (**Table 1.1**). Many of the diseases are immunologically mediated. They may be localized strictly to the joints (e.g., osteoarthritis), or they may have extra-articular and systemic manifestations (e.g., lupus and rheumatoid arthritis).

Table 1.1   Features and Prevalence of Selected Rheumatic Diseases

DISEASE	APPROXIMATE PREVALENCE	RISK FACTORS	AFFECTED ORGANS/JOINTS
Osteoarthritis	10%, increases with age X-ray prevalence >80% over 80 years	Older age Greater Body Mass Index Family history: women with distal interphalangeal and proximal interphalangeal osteoarthritis— Heberden's and Bouchard's nodes Secondary to inflammatory disorders Trauma Heredity (familial osteoarthritis) Metabolic disorders (e.g., hemachromatosis)	Hips, knees, lumbo-sacral spine, hands (distal interphalangeal, proximal inter-phalangeal, first (thumb) carpo-metacarpal joints) weight-bearing joints. Spares metacarpo-phalangeal joints unless secondary to other process
Fibromyalgia	2%; often secondary to other rheumatic diseases	Female-to-male: 9:1 Peak onset: 20–50 years	Muscles, nerves, and soft tissues

(continues)

1

Table 1.1   Features and Prevalence of Selected Rheumatic Diseases, cont'd

Disease	Approximate Prevalence	Risk Factors	Affected Organs/Joints
Rheumatoid arthritis	0.5–1.0%	Female-to-male: 3:1 Smoking Peak onset: 25–55 years Familial predisposition Increased HLA-DR4, HLA-DR1	Hands, metacarpo-phalangeal and proximal interphalangeal joints, wrists, feet (metatarso-phalangeal joints), cervical spine, knees, elbows, shoulders, skin (rheumatoid nodule), lung, vascular (atherosclerosis)
Gout	0.5%	Older age Male (after puberty) Postmenopausal women, diuretic use Cyclosporine use Surgery Alcohol use Rare inherited disorders of urate metabolism (hypoxanthine-guanine phosphoribosyl transferase deficiency and 5-phospho-alpha-d-ribosyl 1-pyrophosphate overactivity, <0.1%)	First metatarso-phalangeal joint, feet, hands, ankles, knees, but any joint may be affected
Pseudogout	0.5% X-ray prevalence >10% over age 70	Female Older age Osteoarthritis Joint trauma Hemochromatosis Hypercalcemia Hyperparathyroidism Hypothyroidism	Wrist, knee, pelvis Radiographs capture >90%

(continues)

Table 1.1   Features and Prevalence of Selected Rheumatic Diseases, cont'd

Disease	Approximate Prevalence	Risk Factors	Affected Organs/Joints
Polymyalgia rheumatica	0.3%	Age >50 European descent	Shoulders, hips, rarely sternoclavicular, knee, wrist joints Proximal stiffness without weakness Giant cell arteritis (estimates vary, but up to 20%)
Ankylosing spondylitis	0.3%	Male-to-female: 3:1 Increased risk in HLA B27 positive individuals Lower risk in African Americans	Spine, sacroiliac joints, peripheral joints (35%), eyes (uveitis) Women sometimes have atypical presentation of neck symptoms before back symptoms
Scleroderma	0.1%	80% female Increased incidence and severity in African Americans	Kidney, lung, digestive system, skin, joints CREST (calcinosis, Raynaud's, esophageal reflux, sclerodactyly, telangectasia)
Psoriatic arthritis	0.1%	Extent of psoriasis not related to extent of arthritis	Fingers (distal interphalangeal joint), toes, "sausage digits," spine, sacroiliac joints, knees, hips, nails, skin, eyes, HIV-associated arthritis
Giant cell arteritis	0.1%	Female-to-male: 3:1 Age >50 European descent	Eyes, temporal arteries, ascending aorta Associated with polymyalgia rheumatica

(continues)

Table 1.1   Features and Prevalence of Selected Rheumatic Diseases, cont'd

Disease	Approximate Prevalence	Risk Factors	Affected Organs/Joints
Systemic lupus erythematosus	0.05%	Female-to-male: 10:1 Non-European descent	Skin, small joints, hematologic symptoms, pericardium, pleura, vascular (atherosclerosis), valvular, pleural, lung, kidney, neuropsychiatric
Dermatomyositis/ polymyositis; inclusion body myositis (IBM)	<0.01%	Female-to-male: 2:1	Proximal muscles, skin, lungs, joints IBM—uniquely distal weakness
Wegener's granulomatosis, vasculitis	<0.01%	30–50 years of age	Lungs, kidneys, head and neck, sinuses, small vessels, peripheral nervous system

The practice of rheumatology is critically dependent on the history and physical examination. In rheumatology, lab results are often more confusing than helpful. Objective diagnostic testing in rheumatology remains rudimentary, and most diagnoses require historical and physical examination features. In fact, the vast majority of diagnostic and management decisions hinge on the clinical history and physical examination, because in many cases a gold standard diagnostic test or disease activity assessment is not easily available. Consequently, diagnoses and management decisions might appear arbitrary and subjective to the novice clinician. The result is that rheumatology can be a particularly difficult discipline to master.

One of the most important distinctions to make in evaluating rheumatologic diseases is to differentiate between inflammatory and noninflammatory conditions. Inflammatory diseases include inflammatory conditions such as rheumatoid arthritis and systemic lupus, crystal diseases, such as gout, pseudogout, and other autoimmune diseases, as well as infectious diseases (see **Table 1.2**). Noninflammatory diseases include a broad range of illnesses that are caused by altered pain perception, mechanical trauma, and repetitive use. The classic non-inflammatory joint disorder is the most common—osteoarthritis.

Table 1.2   Inflammatory Versus Noninflammatory Rheumatologic Diseases

INFLAMMATORY

Infectious Diseases

Septic arthritis, including gonococcal
Tuberculosis arthritis
Fungal arthritis
Lyme disease
Viral arthritis
  Hepatitis B, C
  Parvovirus B19

Crystal Diseases

Gout
Pseudogout (calcium pyrophosphate dihydrate, CPPD)
Apatite deposition

Inflammatory Arthritic Diseases

Rheumatoid arthritis

Spondyloarthropathies
  Psoriatic arthritis
  Ankylosing spondylitis
  Reactive arthritis
  Inflammatory bowel disease (IBD)-associated
Polymyalgia rheumatica

Autoimmune Systemic Diseases with Arthritis Component

Vasculitis
  Wegener's granulomatosis
  Microscopic polyangiitis
  Antineutrophil cytoplasmic antibody (ANCA)-associated
  Immune complex (cryoglobulins, Hepatitis B and C)
  Giant cell artertitis
  Polyarteritis nodosa
  Takayasu's arteritis
  Henoch-Schonlein purpura
Sarcoid
Systemic lupus erythematosus
Still's disease

NONINFLAMMATORY

Osteoarthritis

Hyperflexibility

(continues)

Table 1.2   Inflammatory Versus Noninflammatory Rheumatologic Diseases, cont'd

NONINFLAMMATORY	
Fibromyalgia	

Regional syndromes
  Neck strain
  Epicondylitis
  Carpal tunnel
  Tarsal tunnel
  Rotator cuff tendonitis
	Trochanteric bursitis
	Anserine bursitis
	Prepatellar bursitis
	Plantar fasciitis

Regional structural disease
  Back—herniated disk
  Meniscal disease
  Rotator cuff tendonitis, tear
  Osteonecrosis	

Neurologic Reflex Sympathetic Dystrophy (RSD)	
Joint tumor	

Inflammatory and noninflammatory diseases can be distinguished with a careful history, physical examination, and selected laboratory studies (**Table 1.3**). Systemic symptoms, particularly those of a chronic nature, such as fever and weight loss, can be very suggestive of an inflammatory process. The presence of more than 30 minutes of morning stiffness is particularly suggestive of inflammatory joint disease. Useful questions to ask the patient to elicit a history of inflammatory joint disease include, "What time do you get up in the morning?" and "What time do you feel as well as you feel for that day?" The time difference in the responses is more suggestive of true stiffness and is an accurate reflection of an inflammatory component if greater than 20 to 30 minutes. Joints that demonstrate inflammation with classic symptoms of rubor (redness), dalor (pain), tumor (swelling), and calor (heat) can be particularly helpful. Additional details of the history, physical examination, and laboratory workup are described subsequently.

Table 1.3   Features of Inflammatory and Noninflammatory Diseases

	INFLAMMATORY	NONINFLAMMATORY
History	• No trauma • Diffuse or multifocal symptoms • Morning stiffness • Constitutional symptoms • Skin rashes • Neuropathic symptoms • Recent infection or surgery	• Trauma • Focal symptoms (single joint) • Weight-bearing joints • Joint pain, worsening with use, but no morning stiffness • No constitutional symptoms

(continues)

Table 1.3   Features of Inflammatory and Noninflammatory Diseases, cont'd

	INFLAMMATORY	**NONINFLAMMATORY**
Physical exam	• Fever, hypertension, hypotension • Oral ulcers • Alopecia • Conjunctivitis, iritis • Sinusitis • Single or multiple swollen or warm joints • Raynaud's • Rash • Murmur • Pleural effusion • Pedal edema • Peripheral neuropathy	• Normal vital signs • No warm joints • Pain/symptoms only at the affected joint • Crepitus • Bony hypertrophy • Hyperflexibility • Swollen joint, but no warmth
Laboratory testing	• Elevated inflammatory markers (C-reactive protein, erythrocyte sedimentation rate) • Anemia • Depressed or elevated platelets • Positive blood cultures • Positive hepatitis panels • Abnormal liver function tests • Abnormal creatine phosphokinase, aldolase • Red cells or red cell casts in urine • Proteinuria • Low albumin • Hypercalcemia • Polyclonal gammopathy on serum protein electrophoresis • Positive antinuclear antibodies, rheumatoid factor, anti-cyclic citrullinated peptide antibody, other markers	• Inflammatory markers in the normal range • Normal complete blood count, liver function tests

Key features of several inflammatory noninfectious arthritides are provided in **Table 1.4**.

Table 1.4   Inflammatory Arthritides

DISEASE	**CLINICAL FEATURES**	**EXAM FEATURES AND STUDIES**
Osteoarthritis (noninflammatory)	Gradual onset Pain with use, better with rest Affects weight-bearing joints (knees, hips) and hands (distal interphalangeal and proximal interphalangeal joints)	**Exam:** crepitus, bony deformities, malalignment, non-inflammatory effusions **Radiographs:** weight-bearing films of the knees, asymmetric joint space narrowing, osteophytes, cartilage loss

(continues)

Table 1.4   Inflammatory Arthritides, cont'd

DISEASE	CLINICAL FEATURES	EXAM FEATURES AND STUDIES
Rheumatoid arthritis	Subacute onset Morning stiffness Symmetric Primarily affects small joints of the hands, wrists, feet, but commonly involves most joints in a symmetrical pattern May affect the cervical spine, spares the lumbar spine	**Exam:** swollen, tender, and warm joints; rheumatoid nodules **Radiographs:** osteopenia, symmetrical joint space narrowing, typical erosions **Studies:** anti-cyclic citrullinated peptide antibody (>95% specific)
Systemic lupus erythematosus	Morning stiffness Fatigue Fevers Photosensitivity Facial rash Pleuritic chest pain Symmetric arthritis Headaches Raynaud's (common in all rheumatic diseases) Mouth ulcers Ligamentous laxity in the small joints causing hyperflexibility	**Exam:** palmar erythema, inflamed joints, mouth ulcers, pleural effusions, malar rash **Studies:** urine analysis (often positive for hematuria and proteinuria), dsDNA (>95% specific), antinuclear antibodies (>95% sensitive), leucopenia, thrombocytopenia, hemolytic anemia
Gout/calcium pyrophosphate dehydrate deposition (pseudogout) Apatite	Acute onset (hours) Affects 1 to 5 joints Very painful Associated with alcohol, soft drink, and protein consumption; renal disease; and diuretics Apatite deposition is chronic and similar to osteoarthritis (Milwaukee shoulder) Rarely chronic and can mimic rheumatoid arthritis	**Exam:** swollen, tender, mono- or oligoarthritis; tophi **Radiographs:** rat bite erosions for gout, chondrocalcinosis for pseudogout **Studies:** presence of crystals on aspiration
Ankylosing spondylitis	Back pain at a young age Back pain awakening patient in the second half of the night and causing morning stiffness that improves with use Alternating buttock pain Back pain not improving with rest Inflammatory eye disease	**Radiographs:** Fergusan views of the hips to reveal sacroiliitis; lumbar spine films to reveal squaring and fusion of vertebrate **Studies:** elevated inflammatory markers, HLA B27 positive in over 90%

(continues)

Table 1.4 Inflammatory Arthritides, cont'd

DISEASE	CLINICAL FEATURES	EXAM FEATURES AND STUDIES
Psoriatic arthritis	Psoriasis, typically before but occasionally after onset of arthritis Oligoarthritis Spondylitis "Pseudorheumatoid" arthritis, Distal interphalangeal joint involvement Nail involvement (pitting and onycholysis)	**Exam:** asymmetric oligoarthritis of large joints, digits (dactylitis involving the entire digit), and toes. Unique inflammation of distal interphalangeal joint. Can be associated with spine disease. Sacroiliitis.
Polymyalgia rheumatica	Acute or subacute onset Relatively sudden onset of proximal (hip and/or shoulder) stiffness without weakness Can be associated with giant cell arteritis	**Exam:** restricted shoulders and hips **Studies:** elevated inflammatory markers **Long term:** 5–10% may progress to rheumatoid arthritis

HISTORY

Obtaining a careful history is the most informative aspect of a rheumatologic evaluation. Eliciting several key features from the patient is critical in terms of distinguishing between inflammatory and noninflammatory conditions and building a differential diagnosis.

Pain

Understanding a patient's pain is a particularly challenging issue. Patients often "hurt all over" and have difficulty localizing their pain. However, focusing the patient's history to elucidate specifically what hurts and when is absolutely necessary in order to direct a diagnostic workup. Patients often can identify a specific region or joint that hurts more than others or at least a specific pain that is the most disabling. It is also critical to understand how long the pain has persisted and at what rate it might be worsening. For example, osteoarthritis presents with longstanding and progressive pain, whereas gout tends to occur very acutely and lasts only briefly. When the pain occurs can also be helpful; inflammatory causes of pain tend to be worse with rest and in the morning, whereas noninflammatory causes of pain are typically worse with use. Physicians often use 1–10 scales to assess the level of pain that a patient is feeling, and these scales are sometimes useful to monitor the course of an individual patient. Some characteristic pain patterns include pain at night with pressure at the shoulder or hip (subacromial and greater trochanteric bursitis), pain with weight bearing (lower extremity arthritic pain), pain in the morning that improves with motion (inflammatory joint pain), back pain radiating down the leg that improves with rest and worsens with ambulation (claudication or pseudo-claudication related to spinal stenosis), and diffuse pain in the joints and soft tissues that is persistent and without a clear pattern (fibromyalgia).

Joints

It is very important to identify whether the symptoms are articular (or arthritic) or soft tissue related. This can be confusing, because a wide variety of pains is periarticular. The classic symptoms of joint inflammation—rubor (redness), dalor (pain), tumor (swelling), and calor (heat)—should be specifically evaluated. Joint pain should be apparent with joint use. For example, pain in the distal interphalangeal (DIP) and proximal interphalangeal (PIP) joints might be worse with writing, turning door knobs, or opening jars. Pain in the ankles and knees might be worse with weight bearing and ambulation rather than at rest. Shoulder pain might be worse with abduction or lifting. On exam, the most important feature is to determine if the joint is limited in motion (flexion contracture in any joint signifies prior synovitis or mechanical limitations), swollen, and if synovitis is present. In general, localized pain in a joint is mechanical (osteoarthritis, meniscal tear, etc.) and diffuse joint pain with swelling tends to be more a sign of synovitis, with the caveat that even osteoarthritis can cause some swelling in the joint, as can acute trauma.

Muscle

Muscle symptoms are important to elicit, but they may be confused with arthritic symptoms. Most diseases of the muscle cause little pain but will cause functional impairment and weakness. Location of the weakness, (e.g., distal or proximal muscle groups) can help differentiate the type of myopathy. Distal muscle weakness, such as inclusion body myositis, results in an inability to remove tops of bottles due to reduced grip strength. Proximal muscle weakness, such as that seen with dermatomyositis and polymyositis, results in the inability to stand easily, climb stairs, or rise up off a toilet seat. For an individual patient it is often important to note if they have had an unexplained decrement in a usual activity, such as a golf or bowling score that is worsening for no apparent reason. Individual muscle groups or movements that might be affected are also important to elicit (such as a foot drop or a wrist drop) and can suggest a peripheral neuropathy, indicating vasculitis or nerve entrapment, including herniated disk. In a patient who has severe pain, even mild resistance may cause pain, leading to the impression of weakness. Often this is helped by seeing if the patient can resist motion for even a short period of time, because patients with true weakness will not be able to resist opposing force.

Skin

A wide range of autoimmune diseases can present with rashes. Appropriate identification of the rash can often help with diagnosis (see **Table 1.5**).

Table 1.5 Skin Rashes and Associated Diseases

SKIN RASH	DISEASE	DESCRIPTION
Gottron's rash	Dermatomyositis	An erythematous, scaly eruption occurring in symmetric fashion over the metacarpophalangeal and interphalangeal joints (looks like psoriasis).
Heliotrope rash	Dermatomyositis	Violaceous eruption on the upper eyelids, often with swelling.
Shawl (or V-) sign	Dermatomyositis	Diffuse, flat, erythematous lesion over the chest and shoulders.
Chronic cutaneous lupus erythematosus (discoid lupus)	Discoid lupus	Typically involves face, scalp and ears. Initially erythematous, elevated papules that evolve so that the center of the papule becomes depressed, faded, and atrophic, while the outer rim enlarges and becomes irregular with hyperkeratosis and scarring.
Tophus	Gout	Subcutaneous or intra- or periarticular chalky deposit.
Erythema migrans	Lyme disease	An expanding, flat, painless skin lesion expanding from the site of a tick bite.
Psoriasis	Psoriatic arthritis	Dry patches with scales; occurs especially on the scalp and ears and genitalia and the skin over extensor surfaces. Psoriatic arthritis in particular correlates with nail involvement.
Rheumatoid nodules	Rheumatoid arthritis	Painful subcutaneous nodules that occur at the extensor surface of the elbows, hands, and feet, but may occur elsewhere.
Acute cutaneous lupus erythematosus (malar rash)	Systemic lupus erythematosus	Classic butterfly rash, appearing on the face, often after sun exposure. Not typically scarring. Spares nasolabial folds.
Subacute cutaneous lupus erythematosus	Systemic lupus erythematosus	Local or generalized pruritic rash appearing after sun exposure.
Lupus panniculitis or any panniculitis including erythema nodosum	Systemic lupus erythematosus	Deep nodules beneath the skin.
Still's rash	Still's disease	Evanescent, salmon-colored rash often prominent after warm bath or shower.

(continues)

Table 1.5   Skin Rashes and Associated Diseases, cont'd

Skin Rash	Disease	Description
Livedo reticularis	Vasculitis, antiphospholipid syndrome	A lacy subtle rash, usually on the wrists and knees.
Palpable purpura	Vasculitis	Elevated purpuric rash; does not blanch with pressure. Usually lower extremity more so than upper extremity.

Neurologic Symptoms

Patients with inflammatory and noninflammatory diseases often have neuropathic symptoms. Patient's should be asked about weakness, numbness, or tingling. For example, an L5 radiculopathy causes symptoms along the large toe and the dorsum of the foot (with weakness of the extensor hallicus, but no reflex asymmetry), and an S1 radiculopathy causes symptoms along the lateral foot but with a decreased ankle reflex. Carpal tunnel, which can occur from a noninflammatory cause, such as overuse, diabetes, thyroid disease, or pregnancy, can also occur with inflammatory arthritis. Peripheral neuropathies may be associated with vasculitides, such as polyarteritis; the classic pattern is sporadic loss of individual peripheral nerves in a progressive pattern.

Constitutional Symptoms

Many inflammatory illnesses are associated with fatigue, weight loss, fever, and chills. Patients with Still's disease (classically a "biquotidien" fever), vasculitis, lupus, or sarcoidosis often will present with chronic persistent fevers. However, fever is not a typical presenting symptom of rheumatoid arthritis.

Disability

How limited a patient is by the symptoms he or she describes is a critical factor in the patient's ultimate ability to function. Patients may describe the same symptoms very differently, and getting a sense of what the patient is actually able to do can help to assess disability. The cornerstone of this history is assessing the patient's ability to complete the activities of daily living, such as bathing, using the toilet, transferring out of bed, preparing food, and ambulating. Fibromyalgia, for example, can often present with symptoms that sound particularly concerning, but may not limit the patient's ability to perform activities of daily living.

Classic Review of Systems

A rheumatologic review of symptoms to screen for specific illnesses can be particularly helpful. Key points are summarized in **Table 1.6.**

Table 1.6   Rheumatology Review of Systems

Symptom	Disease
Raynaud's	Systemic lupus erythematosus, rheumatoid arthritis, scleroderma
Mouth ulcers	Systemic lupus erythematosus, Bechet disease
Headaches	Systemic lupus erythematosus, giant cell arteritis, pachymeningitis (secondary to rheumatoid arthritis or other conditions)
Seizures	Systemic lupus erythematosus, CNS vasculitis, anticardiolipin syndromes
Strokes	Antiphospholipid antibody syndrome
Visual disturbances	Giant cell arteritis, systemic lupus erythematosus
Hearing loss	Vasculitis (Wegener's), Cogan's syndrome
Nosebleeds, gingival abnormalities	Systemic lupus erythematosus, idiopathic thrombocytopenic purpura, vasculitis (Wegener's)
Chest pain	Pleuritis secondary to lupus, rheumatoid arthritis, etc.
Acid reflux	Scleroderma, CREST, Raynaud's
Abdominal pain	Lupus—serositis or vasculitis
Edema	Renal disease secondary to vasculitis or lupus
Shortness of breath	Pulmonary fibrosis or interstitial lung disease (scleroderma, rheumatoid arthritis, dermatomyositis, lupus)
Anxiety	Fibromyalgia
Diarrhea	Inflammatory bowel disease, Whipple's disease, celiac sprue

Social History

It is important to elicit a detailed social history. Many aspects of the social history may give clues to the eventual diagnosis, such as exposure to children (parvovirus), activities such as hiking (Lyme disease), smoking (increased incidence of RA), sun exposure (SLE exacerbations), among others. In addition, the patients ability to function in their home and at their workplace may be profoundly affected by their illness, and aggressive intervention with services such as physical and occupational therapies may allow the patients to continue with a relatively normal lifestyle.

Physical Exam

The physical exam is a critical component to diagnosing rheumatologic diseases. This chapter will emphasize the joint exam. In the rheumatologic joint exam, each joint should be evaluated individually. Several general features can be assessed for all joints.

General Appearance

A tremendous amount of information about the joints can be determined by observing the patient prior to the formal exam. The patient's gait can suggest whether lower extremity joints or the feet are involved, and the patient's posture can suggest back involvement. The patient's handshake may suggest disease involvement in the small joints of the hands. The patient's inability to climb onto the gurney might reveal shoulder and hip pathology.

Appearance of the Joint

Simply looking at the joints individually can be helpful. Inflamed joints may appear grossly swollen or even red. Damaged joints will have bony abnormalities toward the end-stage. For example, wrists affected by rheumatoid arthritis are fused, and digits may exhibit ulnar deviation.

Passive Range of Motion

Each joint should be moved individually by the examiner, without assistance from the patient, to assess whether there is any limitation or pain. When passive motion of a joint exceeds active motion, tendon rupture or neurologic involvement, such a herniated disk or nerve injury, must be considered. Limited range of motion may suggest synovial inflammation, an effusion, or a mechanical obstruction. Joints with osteoarthritis may have loose bodies preventing a full range of motion, and meniscal tears in the knee might limit range of motion. A knee effusion will prevent full flexion and full extension altogether, or at the very least be painful. Impingement of the rotator cuff will cause pain with passive external rotation of the shoulder. Chronic joint changes and destruction such as with osteoarthritis or rheumatoid arthritis may result in permanent limitations in range of motion that may not be painful. Adhesive capsulitis presents with limited shoulder abduction. In contrast, individuals with lupus may be hyperflexible and have expanded range of motion if they have the so-called Jaccoud's arthropathy.

Active Range of Motion

The patient should also be asked to move their joints without the help of the examiner. If the patient is more symptomatic when moving the joints on his or her own, it might suggest periarticular structures such as tendons or muscles as opposed to the joint capsule itself. For example, subacromial bursitis may present with completely normal passive shoulder abduction but pain with active shoulder abduction. A torn rotator cuff may present with completely normal passive shoulder abduction but inability to actively abduct the shoulder.

Resisted Movement

To isolate a specific tendon or muscle group, the examiner can fix a joint in a specific position and ask the patient to flex or extend the joint against isometric resistance from the examiner. If pain results, it may suggest a specific muscle, tendon, or muscle group. For example, resisted flexion of the elbow resulting in pain at the shoulder might suggest bicepital tendonitis. Similarly, pain with resisted abduction of the shoulder might suggest rotator cuff tendon disease.

Palpation

Joints should be palpated. Inflamed joints with synovial thickening will have a boggy feel. They may also have more obvious fluid within them, suggesting an effusion that will be more fluctuant. Knee effusions, in particular, can be large and relatively easy to identify by palpation and are a valuable indicator of inflammatory or infectious arthritis or osteoarthritis. A knee effusion will bulge out from under the patella and cause the patella to be ballotable. In addition, a fluid wave may be seen if a knee effusion is present. During palpation, joints should also be assessed for warmth, which would suggest inflammation.

Assessing for Pain During Palpation

During palpation, joints can also be assessed for chronic changes and deformities related to cartilage destruction and joint damage. Specifically, bony changes can often be felt directly, and crepitus might be appreciated if there is cartilage destruction. While palpating the joint, it is important to assess whether specific structures might be painful. For example, anserine bursitis results in pain with palpation of the medial-inferior aspect of the tibial plateau. Trochanteric bursitis results in pain with palpation of the lateral hip over the trochanter. Subacromial bursitis results in pain with palpation of the lateral aspect of the affected shoulder. Fibromyalgia results in pain with palpation of periarticular structures. Inflamed joints are often diffusely painful.

JOINT ASPIRATION

A critical aspect of a rheumatologic evaluation is a joint aspiration. For patents presenting with an acute monoarthritis, where septic arthritis is on the differential diagnosis, a joint aspiration is an absolutely necessary element of the initial evaluation. Even in cases where infectious arthritis is not a consideration, a joint aspiration is most helpful in distinguishing inflammatory from noninflammatory diseases. Many joints, such as the knee, ankle, wrist, and elbow, are easily aspirated at the bedside. Shoulder and hip aspirations typically require guidance by ultrasound or computed tomography (**Table 1.7**).

Table 1.7   Joint Aspiration

DISEASE	CRYSTAL	CELL COUNT, DIFFERENTIAL
Noninflammatory osteoarthritis	N/A	<1500 wbc/mm³ (<25% Polys)
Autoimmune/inflammatory arthritis	N/A	1500–50,000 wbc/mm³ (>50% Polys) Rarely up to 100,000 wbc/mm³
Crystalline arthritis —pseudogout	CPPD (dull, rhomboid-shaped, intracellular, positive birefringence)	1000–50,000 mm³ (>50% Polys) Presence of crystals does not rule out infection—may coexist
Crystalline arthritis—gout	Uric acid (bright, needle-shaped, intracellular, negative birefringence)	1000–50,000 wbc mm³ (>50% Polys) Presence of crystals does not rule out infection—may coexist
Infectious arthritis	N/A	>50,000 wbc/mm³ (>75% Polys Joint white counts as low as 1000 may occur in immunocompromised patients, and in patients with tuberculosis and gonococcus among others

SUMMARY

This chapter summarized the essential ingredients of the initial accounter with a patient who presents with rheumatologic symptoms. The most important differential for the clinician is to determine if the patient has an inflammatory disorder. This determination is the main branch point for further evaluation. If it is determined that the presenting symptoms are not inflammatory, then there is a totally different differential diagnosis to consider.

Local conditions predominate for nonsystemic illnesses, and these include regional disorders as well as osteoarthritis and neck and/or back pain. If the signs point to an inflammatory condition, then there is another unique set of differential diagnostic entities to consider—from rheumatoid arthritis to systemic lupus erythematosus (SLE). It is hoped that this book will help the practitioner differentiate between inflammatory and noninflammatory conditions and then decide how to further evaluate and subsequently treat the patient.

◇◇◇◇◇◇◇◇◇◇◇◇◇◇◇◇◇◇◇◇

SUGGESTED READINGS

Alguire PC, Epstein PE, American College of Physicians. *MKSAP 14: Medical knowledge self-assessment program. Part A.* Philadelphia: American College of Physicians; 2006.

American College of Rheumatology. High impact rheumatology curriculum; 2009. Available at: http://www.rheumatology.org/educ/hir/ppt.asp.

American College of Rheumatology Ad Hoc Committee on Clinical Guidelines. Guidelines for the initial evaluation of the adult patient with acute musculoskeletal symptoms. *Arthritis Rheum.* 1996;39(1):1–8.

Fam AG, Lawry GV, Kreder HJ. *Musculoskeletal examination and joint injection techniques.* Philadelphia: Mosby/Elsevier; 2006.

Harris ED, Ruddy S, Kelley WN. *Kelley's textbook of rheumatology.* 7th ed. Philadelphia: Elsevier Saunders; 2005.

Harrison TR, Fauci AS, Langford CA. *Harrison's rheumatology.* New York: McGraw-Hill; 2006.

Hochberg MC. *Rheumatology.* 4th ed. Philadelphia: Mosby/Elsevier; 2008.

Isenberg D. *Oxford textbook of rheumatology.* 3rd ed. New York: Oxford University Press; 2004.

Polley HF, Hunder GG, Beetham WP. *Rheumatologic interviewing and physical examination of the joints.* 2d ed. Philadelphia: Saunders; 1978.

CHAPTER 2

Laboratory Tests in Rheumatology

Thorvardur Jon Love, MD

OVERVIEW

Laboratory tests in rheumatology can be divided into three main categories: nonspecific measures of inflammation, markers of end-organ involvement, and autoantibodies suggestive of an individual disease or group of diseases.

The first category includes inflammatory markers commonly used in clinical practice, such as the erythrocyte sedimentation rate (ESR) and the C-reactive protein (CRP). Experimental inflammatory markers include interleukin-6 (IL-6) and tumor necrosis factor-alpha (TNF-alpha). These laboratory tests can be used to detect inflammation when it is not clinically obvious, and in some cases follow disease activity over time. However, they are not diagnostic of a particular disease nor are they specific to rheumatologic diseases, because infections, malignancies, and other disorders can also increase their levels.

The second category refers to changes in laboratory tests such as liver function tests, blood counts, and renal function tests that may signal disease involvement of particular organ systems.

The third category encompasses the autoantibodies produced in a number of autoimmune disorders, but their sensitivity and specificity vary. Examples of these autoantibodies include the rheumatoid factor (RF), anti-cyclic citrullinated protein (aCCP), and antinuclear antibodies (ANA). When used in the appropriate clinical setting, specific autoantibodies can be helpful in confirming the diagnosis of autoimmune diseases. However, these tests must be interpreted carefully, because they can be found in the general population and their significance depends on the prior probability of disease. Therefore, they should not be used as a general screen in persons who do not have symptoms or signs suggestive of a particular rheumatologic disorder.

MARKERS OF INFLAMMATION

Of the inflammatory markers, the oldest and best known is the erythrocyte sedimentation rate (ESR), which was first described in 1897.[1] The Westergren method is used most commonly. Red blood cells are placed in an upright tube and their rate of sedimentation is measured in mm/hr. This rate of sedimentation is influenced by how readily red blood cells cluster, which, in turn, is influenced by the presence of byproducts of inflammation in the bloodstream, primarily fibrinogen and immunoglobulin. It is therefore a nonspecific measure of inflammation of any cause. The ESR rises with age in normal individuals, and therefore the normal value should be adjusted for age using the following formula:[2]

Upper limit of normal ESR = Age (+10 if Female)/2

The ESR can be elevated in any autoimmune disease, but in rheumatology very high values of 100 or more are most commonly thought of in association with polymyalgia rheumatica (PMR) and giant cell arteritis (GCA). Although it is often measured as part of a rheumatology workup, the ESR may be elevated in any inflammatory condition. The most common causes of an ESR of 100 or more are infection (33%), malignancy (17%), and renal disease (17%), with only 14% being from autoimmune disorders.[3] Therefore, the relevance of an elevated ESR must be interpreted in the setting of other clinical evidence. Other conditions that may increase the sedimentation rate include some anemias and pregnancy.

The C-reactive protein (CRP) takes its name from the fact that it reacts with the C-polysaccharide on bacteria. It rises and falls faster with changes in inflammatory activity than the ESR. The maximum ESR value is limited by the length of the Westergren tube (usually 120 mm), but the CRP has no upper limit. Cigarette smoking, obesity, diabetes, and pregnancy may also elevate the CRP, although the latter has more of an impact on the ESR.[4–6]

The ESR and CRP are commonly used to monitor disease activity and help evaluate the clinical response to therapeutic agents. Although the fast response and wider range of the CRP may seem to make it more suitable for testing for inflammation, the two tests are in fact complementary, because one may be elevated when the other is not. It is therefore advisable to check both when initially evaluating a patient for inflammation and then use the one that seems to track more closely with clinical disease activity for monitoring. Inflammatory markers such as IL-6 and anti-TNF are used in research and may be available in some clinical laboratories, but their role in clinical practice has not been defined.

GENERAL LABORATORY STUDIES IN RHEUMATOLOGIC DISORDERS

In addition to specific autoantibodies and nonspecific markers of inflammation, some autoimmune diseases cause changes in laboratory values that suggest organ involvement. For example, the most useful lab test when a patient is suspected of having polymyositis (PM) or dermatomyositis (DM) is the creatinine kinase (CK), which is almost always elevated. Aldolase, aspartate aminotransferase (AST), and alanine aminotransferase (ALT) are often elevated as well, and the latter two may lead to the mistaken diagnosis of liver disease, when in fact they originate in muscle, whereas aldolase may be elevated due to hemolysis or liver disease.

Table 2.1 lists some blood studies commonly evaluated in clinical practice and their relationship to a selection of autoimmune diseases. These findings are not universally present, but when they are they can lend supportive data to the diagnosis of the disorder.

Table 2.1   Changes in Laboratory Values Associated with Autoimmune Disorders

	RHEUMATOID ARTHRITIS	SYSTEMIC LUPUS ERYTHEMATOSUS	POLYMYOSITIS OR DERMATO-MYOSITIS	GIANT CELL ARTERITIS	POLYMYALGIA RHEUMATICA	VASCULITIS**
White blood cell	↔	↓	↔	↔	↔	↔
Hemoglobin/ hematocrit	↓	↓	↔	↓	↔↓	↔↓
Platelets		↓	↔		↔	
AST and ALT	↔	↔			↔	↔
Albumin	↓	↔	↔	↓	↔	↔
CK	↔	↔		↔	↔	↔
Aldolase	↔	↔	↑	↔	↔	↔
Creatinine	↔	*	↔	↔	↔	↔

↑ = high, ↓ = low, ↔ = unchanged.
 * Creatinine may be elevated in SLE-associated renal disease.
 ** Changes in vasculitis depend on the organ involved.

COMPLEMENTS

Although not a specific marker of any single disease, complement levels can be a useful marker of disease activity. They are usually evaluated by measuring CH50, which evaluates the functional integrity of the classical pathway using diluted serum and antibody-coated sheep red blood cells, as well as by checking the C3 and C4 levels directly by enzyme-linked immunosorbant assay (ELISA). Any rheumatic disease that results in immune complex deposition may result in lowered complement levels, but the two best known examples are systemic lupus erythematosus (SLE) and cryoglobulinemia. Certain congenital complement deficiencies, including low or deficient C1q, C1r, C1s, C2, C3, and C4, are associated with SLE or SLE-like illness. Complement levels offer different information than the ESR and CRP, because they tend to be elevated in infections where the production of new complements can keep pace with consumption but are depressed in disease states associated with immune complex deposition and consequent complement consumption. Notable exceptions from this rule are subacute bacterial endocarditis (SBE) and poststreptococcal glomerulonephritis, both of which can depress complement levels. **Table 2.2** shows examples of conditions associated with low and normal/elevated complement levels.

Table 2.2   Complement Levels in Various Conditions

Low	Normal or Elevated
Systemic lupus erythematosus	Infection*
Mixed cryoglobulinemia	Inflammatory conditions (e.g. rheumatoid
Serum sickness	arthritis, spondyloarthopathies)
Vasculitis (some—not always)	Pregnancy
Postinfectious glomerulonephritis	
Congenital complement deficiencies	

*Exceptions: Subacute bacterial endocarditis, postinfectious glomerulonephritis.
Adapted from UpToDate, www.uptodate.com.

RHEUMATOID FACTOR (RF) AND ANTI-CYCLIC CITRULLINATED PEPTIDE (ACCP)

Probably the best known autoantibody in rheumatology is the rheumatoid factor (RF). It is an antibody against the Fc portion of IgG antibodies. Although studies have reported that in cohorts of patients with rheumatoid arthritis the prevalence of RF can be upwards of 80%,[7] population-based studies suggest a lower prevalence of RF in rheumatoid arthritis of 26 to 60%.[8–11] Of note, it can be positive in 4% of the normal population at large and in 25% of the older population. Therefore, it is unsuitable as a screening tool, because 90% of RF-positive individuals will not have rheumatoid arthritis and as many as 80% may convert back to seronegative status over a period of a few years.[12] In addition to rheumatoid arthritis, RF can be positive in SLE, Sjögren's syndrome, mixed cryoglobulinemia, chronic liver disease (most commonly hepatitis C), Lyme disease, SBE, and tuberculosis. Because some of these conditions can cause arthritis independent of rheumatoid arthritis, they should be part of the differential diagnosis when evaluating a positive RF.

The anti-cyclic citrullinated peptide (aCCP) is an ELISA assay that detects antibodies to cyclic citrullinated peptides. It was developed in 2000 following the discovery of anti-citrullinated protein antibodies in rheumatoid arthritis patients.[13] It is more specific than RF for rheumatoid arthritis (95% vs. 85%), with similar sensitivity (67% vs. 69%).[14]

When choosing laboratory tests for a patient with symptoms consistent with rheumatoid arthritis, it may be useful to check both the RF and the aCCP, because 34% of rheumatoid arthritis patients with a negative RF have a positive aCCP.

ANTINUCLEAR ANTIBODIES (ANA)

The test for antinuclear antibodies (ANA) may be performed in one or two steps, depending on the laboratory. Many laboratories use an ELISA to screen for ANA before using immunofluorescence on a cell substrate to confirm the titer and pattern, whereas other labs will go directly to the cell-substrate test. The substrate for immunofluorescence used to be mouse liver cells, but now a human Hep-2 cell line is most often used. The test detects any antibodies directed against the cell nucleus. In addition to a titer, a pattern of nuclear staining can be described.

Although ANA are commonly associated with SLE, they are seen in many other autoimmune disorders, as well as in the general population. ANA is positive in 92 to 98% of all patients with SLE and in up to 30% of the normal population at the level of 1:40 and 13% of the population at 1:80.[15] Thus, a positive ANA does not make the diagnosis of SLE. However, it is highly unlikely that an individual has SLE in the absence of a positive ANA. ANA results are reported as a titer, starting at 1/40 and going to 1/80, 1/160, 1/320, and so on. If the ANA is in the 1/40 to 1/160 range, it is considered borderline; correspondingly, the range of ANA positivity in the healthy population is 5 to 32%. However, a level of 1/320 is usually considered positive, being found in only 3% of the healthy population, and may warrant evaluation.[15]

Another useful feature of the ANA is the staining pattern, which can be homogenous, diffuse, speckled, centromeric, peripheral, or nucleolar. These staining patterns usually reflect which specific antinuclear antibodies have given rise to the positive ANA screen. **Table 2.3** shows how different staining patterns are associated with underlying nuclear antibodies, as well as their disease associations.

Table 2.3   ANA Staining Patterns, Underlying Nuclear Antigens, and Disease Associations

STAINING PATTERN	NUCLEAR ANTIGENS	ASSOCIATION
Homogenous / Diffuse	dsDNA	SLE
	Histone	SLE, drug-induced disease
Peripheral / Rim	dsDNA	SLE
Speckled	Smith, RNP	SLE, mixed connective tissue disease
	SSA(Ro)/SSB(La)	SLE, Sjögren's
Centromeric	Centromere	CREST/limited sclerosis
Nucleolar	RNA	Scleroderma

The specific ANA most commonly associated with SLE are anti-smith and the anti-double-stranded DNA (dsDNA). The antihistone antibody is associated with drug-induced lupus and a homogenous ANA pattern.

ANTIBODIES FOUND IN THE INFLAMMATORY MYOPATHIES

Autoantibodies are found in up to 80% of patients with PM/DM, and some of them are associated with distinct clinical patterns.[16,17] Because 20% of patients with PM/DM have no detectable autoantibodies, these are not required for diagnosis in the appropriate clinical setting. **Table 2.4** lists the most common autoantibodies found in PM/DM and their association with clinical patterns and prognosis.

Table 2.4   Antigens Against Which Antibodies Are Found in Myositis and Their Clinical Correlations and Frequencies

Antigen	Frequency in Myositis	Correlation
Any nuclear (ANA) RNP/Scl-70	70–80%	Nonspecific MCTD/scleroderma
Jo-1, OJ, EJ, PL-7, PL-12	20–30%, combined	Antisynthetase syndrome (Raynaud's, interstitial lung disease (ILD), arthritis, mechanic's hands)
Mi-2	5–10%	DM
SRP	5%	PM (poor prognosis)
Exosome complex (PM/Scl)		PM and scleroderma overlap

ANTIBODIES ASSOCIATED WITH SCLERODERMA

Autoantibodies are found in at least 70% of patients with scleroderma and can be used to identify clinical subgroups with important prognostic implications.[18] Because 30% of patients with scleroderma have no autoantibodies, these are not required for diagnosis in the appropriate clinical setting. **Table 2.5** lists the major autoantibodies associated with scleroderma and their clinical correlations.

Table 2.5   Major Antibodies Found in Scleroderma and Their Clinical Significance

Antibody	Clinical Significance
ANA (centromere pattern)	Limited sclerosis, CREST, pulmonary hypertension, primary biliary cirrhosis, relatively good prognosis
Anti-RNA polymerase	Diffuse sclerosis, scleroderma, renal crisis, poor prognosis

(continues)

Table 2.5   Major Antibodies Found in Scleroderma and Their Clinical Significance, cont'd

ANTIBODY	CLINICAL SIGNIFICANCE
Anti-Scl-70	Diffuse sclerosis, pulmonary disease, poor prognosis
Anti-U1-RNP	Mixed connective tissue disease with scleroderma
Anti-U3-RNP	Pulmonary hypertension with scleroderma

Adapted from UpToDate, www.uptodate.com.

MIXED CONNECTIVE TISSUE DISEASE (MCTD) AND OVERLAP SYNDROMES

Mixed connective tissue disease (MCTD) shares autoantibodies with other rheumatic conditions, and more than 50% of MCTD patients have a positive RF. The diagnosis of MCTD rests on the presence of anti-U1-RNP antibody.[19] However, this autoantibody is not entirely specific for MCTD, because it is present in undifferentiated connective tissue disease as well as other rheumatic diseases.

Other overlap disorders, where patients exhibit features of more than one rheumatic disease, can be associated with autoantibodies specific for multiple rheumatic diseases. No specific autoantibody identifies these overlap syndromes, with the exception of anti-PM/Scl in the overlap of polymyositis and scleroderma.[20]

ANTIPHOSPHOLIPID ANTIBODIES

Antiphospholipid antibodies are antibodies that are directed against phospholipids. They are associated with antiphospholipid syndrome, which is marked by arterial clotting events, venous clotting events, and obstetric complications. Other features are discussed elsewhere. The antibodies are not specific to this disorder, because 1 to 5% of the general population has these antibodies and an even greater proportion are seen in other patient groups, in particular after infections.[21] The diagnosis of antiphospholipid syndrome requires clinical features in addition to laboratory testing, and treatment is only indicated in those with history of clotting. The first described antiphospholipid antibody was a false-positive Venereal Disease Research Laboratory (VDRL) test and rapid plasma reagin (RPR), reflecting the nonspecific activity of the sera against the cardiolipin that is used in this assay. The more specific tests are the lupus anticoagulant (LAC) and the anticardiolipin antibodies (ACA). The name of the former test is misleading, because it is not always associated with lupus and it is a procoagulant in vivo. The initial test varies from lab to lab but can include any prolongation of a clotting test. Commonly used tests include an activated partial thromboplastin time (aPTT), dilute Russell viper venom time (RVVT), kaolin clotting time, and others. If the initial screen is positive, then a two-step confirmatory test is done. First, normal sera is added back to see if the clotting prolongation corrects. If it does, it suggests the presence of a factor deficiency. If, however, the clotting test is still prolonged, then phospholipids are added to the test to see if it corrects the lupus anticoagulant. True positive testing is only confirmed after this two-step confirmatory evaluation is performed.

The other antiphospholipid antibody is an IgG or IgM anti-anticardiolipin antibody or, less commonly, an antibody against beta-2-glycoprotein-1. These antibodies are detected using a fluorescent ELISA assay, allowing for high sensitivity, but separate assays are needed for each antibody, as well as their subtypes. Although other subtypes of these antibodies have been found (e.g., IgA and IgD), for the purposes of diagnosis only the IgM and IgG subtypes are recognized.

ANTINEUTROPHIL CYTOPLASM ANTIBODIES (ANCA)

Antineutrophil cytoplasm antibodies (ANCA) were first described as being associated with vasculitis in the 1980s. ANCA is tested for in two stages. First, a screen is performed using a sensitive immunofluorescent test, and if the screen is positive an ELISA is used to determine the ANCA subtype. Two staining patterns are detectable on the screening test, which correlate with the ELISA subtypes. The cytoplasmic (c-ANCA) pattern is usually associated with antiproteinase 3 (anti-PR3) on the ELISA test, and the perinuclear (p-ANCA) pattern usually predicts a positive ELISA for antimyeloperoxidase activity (anti-MPO). **Table 2.6** lists the ANCA antibodies and their associations with different vasculitidies.

Table 2.6   ANCA Frequency by Disease and Underlying Antigens

DISEASE	ANCA+	PR3	MPO
Generalized WG	90%	80–85%	10%
Limited WG	40–50%	Mostly PR3	
MPA	75%	5–10%	60–70%
CSS	50%		More often MPO
Anti-GBM	10–40%		Mostly MPO
Classic PAN, GCA	0%		

WG = Wegener's granulomatosis
MPA = Microscopic polyangiitis
CSS = Churg-Strauss Syndrome
GBM = Glomerular Basement Membrane

◇◇◇◇◇◇◇◇◇◇◇◇

REFERENCES

1. Biernacki E. Samoistna sedymentacja krwi jako naukowa, praktyczno-kliniczna metoda badania. *Gazeta Lekarska.* 1897;17:962, 996.

2. Miller A, Green M, Robinson D. Simple rule for calculating normal erythrocyte sedimentation rate. *Br Med J (Clin Res Ed).* 1983;286(6361):266.

3. Fincher RM, Page MI. Clinical significance of extreme elevation of the erythrocyte sedimentation rate. *Arch Intern Med.* 1986;146(8):1581–1583.

4. Ford ES. Body mass index, diabetes, and C-reactive protein among U.S. adults. *Diabetes Care.* 1999;22(12):1971–1977.

5. Ohsawa M, Okayama A, Nakamura M, et al. CRP levels are elevated in smokers but unrelated to the number of cigarettes and are decreased by long-term smoking cessation in male smokers. *Prev Med.* 2005;41(2):651–656.

6. Sacks GP, Seyani L, Lavery S, Trew G. Maternal C-reactive protein levels are raised at 4 weeks gestation. *Hum Reprod.* 2004;19(4):1025–1030.

7. Wolfe F, Cathey MA, Roberts FK. The latex test revisited. Rheumatoid factor testing in 8,287 rheumatic disease patients. *Arthritis Rheum.* 1991;34(8): 951–960.

8. Kellgren JH. Epidemiology of rheumatoid arthritis. *Arthritis Rheum.* 1966;9(5):658–674.

9. Mikkelsen WM, Dodge HJ, Duff IF, Kato H. Estimates of the prevalence of rheumatic diseases in the population of Tecumseh, Michigan, 1959–1960. *J Chronic Dis.* 1967;20(6): 351–369.

10. Cathcart ES, O'Sullivan JB. Rheumatoid arthritis in a New England town. A prevalence study in Sudbury, Massachusetts. *N Engl J Med.* 1970;282(8):421–424.

11. Lichtenstein MJ, Pincus T. Rheumatoid arthritis identified in population based cross sectional studies: low prevalence of rheumatoid factor. *J Rheumatol.* 1991;18(7):989–993.

12. Gran JT, Johannessen A, Husby G. A study of IgM rheumatoid factors in a middle-aged population of Northern Norway. *Clin Rheumatol.* 1984;3(2):163–168.

13. Schellekens GA, Visser H, de Jong BA, et al. The diagnostic properties of rheumatoid arthritis antibodies recognizing a cyclic citrullinated peptide. *Arthritis Rheum.* 2000;43(1):155–163.

14. Nishimura K, Sugiyama D, Kogata Y, et al. Meta-analysis: diagnostic accuracy of anti-cyclic citrullinated peptide antibody and rheumatoid factor for rheumatoid arthritis. *Ann Intern Med.* 2007;146(11):797–808.

15. Tan EM, Feltkamp TE, Smolen JS, et al. Range of antinuclear antibodies in "healthy" individuals. *Arthritis Rheum.* 1997;40(9):1601–1611.

16. Reichlin M, Arnett, FC Jr. Multiplicity of antibodies in myositis sera. *Arthritis Rheum.* 1984;27(10):1150–1156.

17. Drake LA, Dinehart SM, Farmer ER, et al. Guidelines of care for dermatomyositis. *J Am Acad Dermatol.*1996;34(5 Pt 1):824–829.

18. Steen VD. Autoantibodies in systemic sclerosis. *Semin Arthritis Rheum.* 2005;35(1):35–42.

19. Alarcon-Segovia D, Cardiel MH. Comparison between 3 diagnostic criteria for mixed connective tissue disease. Study of 593 patients. *J Rheumatol.* 1989;16(3):328–334.

20. Oddis CV, Okano Y, Rudert WA, Trucco M, Duquesnoy RJ, Medsger TA Jr. Serum autoantibody to the nucleolar antigen PM-Scl. Clinical and immunogenetic associations. *Arthritis Rheum.* 1992;35(10):1211–1217.

21. Vlachoyiannopoulos PG, Samarkos M, Sikara M, Tsiligros P. Antiphospholipid antibodies: laboratory and pathogenetic aspects. *Crit Rev Clin Lab Sci.* 2007;44(3):271–338.

CHAPTER 3

Bone Radiology

Roger Han, MD

OVERVIEW

Radiographs are a common technique for evaluating rheumatologic conditions. They can aid in diagnosis, help determine disease severity, and monitor disease progression. Multiple factors must be considered when analyzing radiographs for arthritic conditions. The primary radiographic considerations are multiple, and include the location and assessment of erosive versus productive features. Other attributes that should be evaluated include joint alignment, bone density, cartilage space, and soft tissues. These latter attributes are more subtle but some (ostepenia) may be the initial finding in a patient with inflammatory joint disease.

RADIOGRAPH EVALUATION

Arthritic processes typically involve specific joints and locations within individual joints and may have a pattern of symmetry across the body. For example, the characteristic distribution of osteoarthritis is involvement of the distal interphalangeal joints, whereas rheumatoid arthritis frequently involves the metacarpophalangeal joints.

Arthropathies also have characteristic patterns of destruction of normal osseous structure (erosions) or production of new bone (osteophytes). Rheumatoid arthritis is the most common purely erosive arthritis. The initial erosions in rheumatoid arthritis are seen at the margins of the joints where there are bare areas of bone that are within the joint capsule but that do not have overlying cartilage. In contrast, osteoarthritis is the most common productive arthritis. Many other arthropathies exhibit a combination of erosive and productive changes, often in typical patterns. The locations of joint changes as well as the type of changes need to be considered in order to arrive at a diagnosis.

Joint alignment is an important attribute in evaluating radiographs. In a neutral, nonstressed position, the articular surfaces of the bones of a joint should be centered on each other. Osseous alignment may be affected in arthropathies by ligamentous laxity or by destructive joint changes. When the articular surface of one bone only partly opposes the other, subluxation occurs. One example of subluxation is volar and ulnar subluxation of the metacarpophalangeal joints seen in late rheumatoid arthritis. Dislocation of a joint can occur when the articular surfaces are entirely out of contact.

Bone density should be evaluated carefully. Inflammatory arthropathies cause hyperemia within the adjacent bones. The relative increased blood flow near the joints causes increased resorption of the mineral matrix of the bone, resulting in relative para-articular osteopenia. On radiographs, osteopenia is manifested by darker bones appearing more like the soft tissues in terms of density.

The thickness of the cartilage spaces needs to be carefully evaluated for narrowing of the space, indicating destruction of the cartilage. The cartilage space of an individual joint should have a uniform thickness across its entire surface. In similar joints, such as the first through fifth metacarpophalangeal joints, the cartilage spaces are normally similar in thickness.

Finally, the soft tissues should be examined carefully for any abnormalities. For example, swelling of the soft tissue of an entire digit is suggestive of psoriatic arthritis ("the sausage digit"), whereas soft tissue nodules can be seen in rheumatoid arthritis.

Radiographs are one of the most useful tools for evaluating arthritic conditions. ABCDES is an easy mnemonic to remember when evaluating a radiograph: Alignment, Bone density, Cartilage, Distribution, Erosions (and productive changes), and Soft tissue.

A simple radiograph is a very useful and cost-effective tool. The radiographs presented here review the essentials of bone radiology in patients with known disease states and offer an elementary summary of the important features of bone radiology.

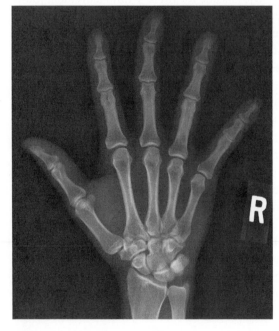

Figure 3.1   Normal hand

Note the normal alignment, bone mineral density, cartilage spaces, normal distribution (lack of symmetric or asymmetric findings), lack of erosions, and normal soft tissues (ABCDES).

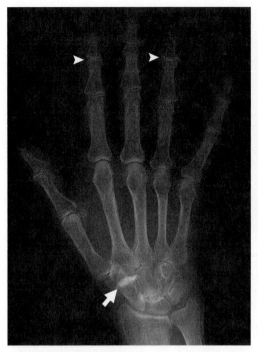

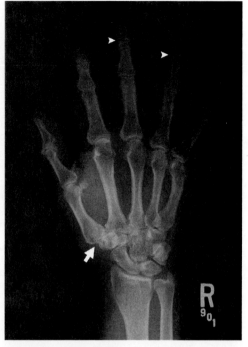

Figure 3.2 Osteoarthritis

This PA radiograph of the hand demonstrates cartilage space narrowing and osteophyte formation at the scaphoid-trapezium-trapezoid joint (arrow) and at the distal interphalangeal joints (arrowheads).

Figure 3.3 Osteoarthritis

This PA view of the hand demonstrates cartilage space narrowing of the distal interphalangeal joints with marginal osteophytes and subchondral cystic changes (arrowheads). Cartilage space narrowing of the first carpometacarpal joint with subchondral cystic changes and osteophytes are also seen (arrow). This is a typical distribution of joint involvement in the hand in osteoarthritis.

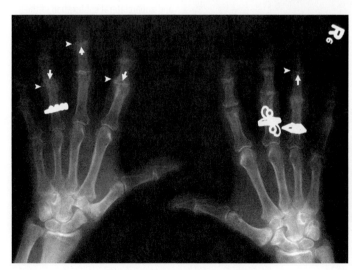

Figure 3.4 Erosive osteoarthritis

Central erosive changes at multiple distal interphalangeal and proximal interphalangeal joints (arrows) with marginal osteophytes (arrowheads), resulting in the characteristic "gull-wing" configuration of the involved interphalangeal joints.

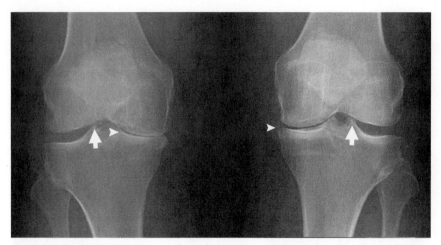

Figure 3.5   Osteoarthritis

This AP radiograph of the knees shows bilateral medial compartment cartilage space narrowing (arrowheads), marginal osteophytes, and tibial spine osteophytes (arrows). The medial compartment of the tibiofemoral joint is the most commonly involved compartment in osteoarthritis.

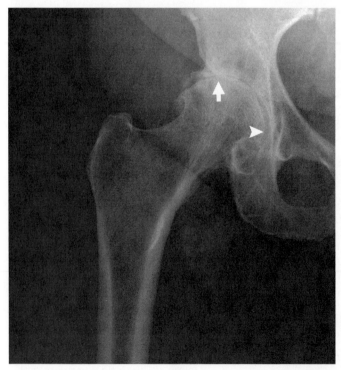

Figure 3.6   Osteoarthritis

This AP radiograph of the hip demonstrates cartilage space narrowing superiorly at the weight-bearing portion of the hip, with relative preservation of the medial cartilage space. Additionally, osteophytes, subchondral sclerosis, buttressing of the femoral neck with increased prominence of the trabecular bone, and superolateral subluxation of the femoral head are demonstrated.

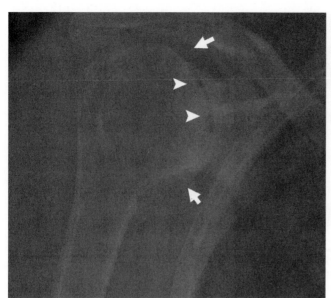

Figure 3.7   Osteoarthritis

This AP view of the shoulder with internal rotation demonstrates full-thickness loss of cartilage space with bone-on-bone appearance, subchondral cystic changes and sclerosis (arrowheads), and a rim of osteophytes at the glenoid and humeral head (arrows).

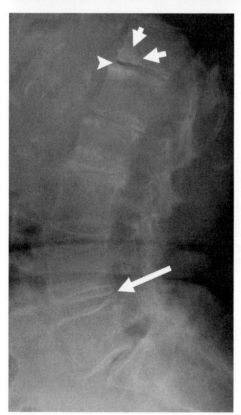

Figure 3.8   Osteoarthritis

This lateral view of the spine shows loss of intervertebral disc height at multiple levels, vacuum phenomenon characterized by gas density within the disc space (arrowhead), and reactive endplate sclerosis forming a triangular area of sclerosis at the anterior margin of the vertebral body (short arrow). In comparison, the L4–L5 disc space is normal, without vacuum phenomenon or endplate sclerosis (long arrow).

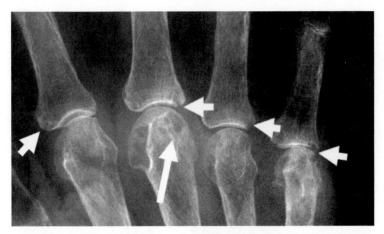

Figure 3.9   Rheumatoid arthritis

This PA radiograph of the metacarpophalangeal joints demonstrates cartilage space narrowing, periarticular osteopenia, marginal erosions of the proximal phalanges (short arrows), and an erosion of the head of the third metacarpal (long arrow).

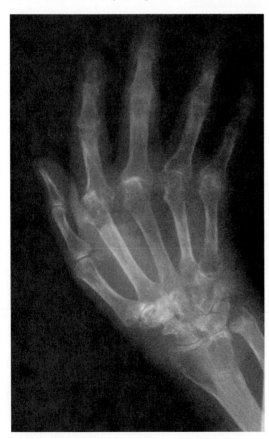

Figure 3.10   Rheumatoid arthritis

This PA radiograph of the hand and wrist demonstrate findings of rheumatoid arthritis, including ulnar deviation of the carpus, volar subluxation and ulnar deviation of the metacarpophalangeal joints, erosion at the ulnar styloid and distal radioulnar joint, and periarticular osteopenia.

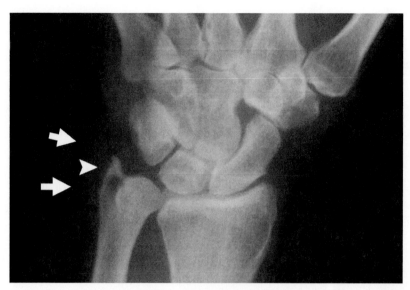

Figure 3.11 Rheumatoid arthritis

This PA radiograph of the wrist demonstrates early findings of rheumatoid arthritis, including erosion of the ulnar styloid (arrowhead) and soft tissue swelling at the ulnar styloid (arrows).

**Figure 3.12
Rheumatoid arthritis**

This lateral view of the calcaneus demonstrates erosions at the posterior calcaneus and soft tissue swelling and inflammatory changes within Keger's fat pad anterior to the Achilles tendon (arrowhead) and the retrocalcaneal bursa (arrows).

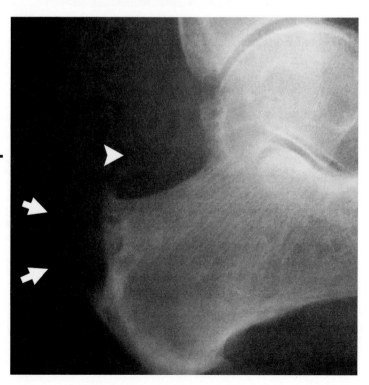

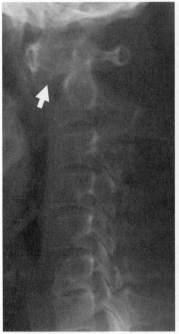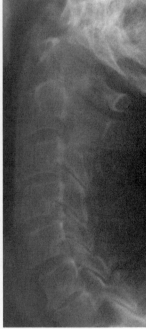

Figure 3.13   Rheumatoid arthritis

Lateral flexion (left) and extension (right) radiographs of the cervical spine demonstrate atlantoaxial subluxation, with widening of the interval between the anterior arch of C1 and the odontoid process on the flexion radiograph (arrow), and normalization of the atlantoaxial interval on the extension radiograph.

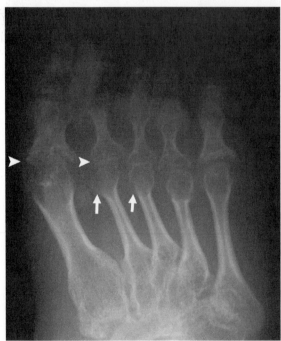

Figure 3.14   Juvenile rheumatoid arthritis

This AP radiograph of the foot demonstrates enlarged epiphyses and metaphyses of the metatarsal heads relative to the diaphyses (arrows) and erosive changes and loss of cartilage space (arrowheads). Overgrowth of the epiphyses and metaphyses occurred due to hyperemia while the patient was skeletally immature, which increased the pace of skeletal maturation.

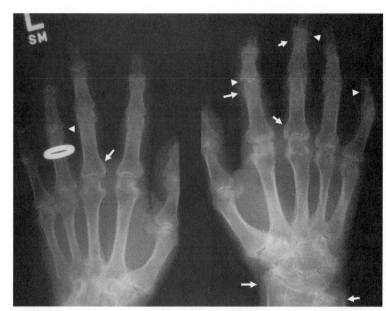

Figure 3.15
Psoriatic arthritis

This PA radiograph of both hands shows marginal erosions at multiple joints (arrowheads), fluffy periostitis near multiple joints, as well as the radial and ulnar styloids (arrows).

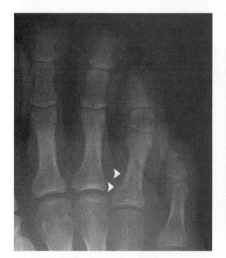

Figure 3.16   Psoriatic arthritis

This AP radiograph of the foot shows diffuse soft tissue swelling of the fourth digit, or "sausage digit," with fluffy periostitis of the proximal phalanx (arrowheads).

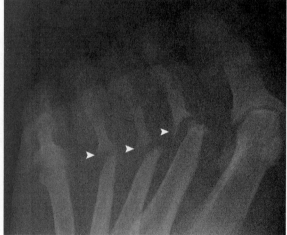

Figure 3.17   Psoriatic arthritis

This AP radiograph of the foot reveals changes of advanced psoriatic arthritis, with erosions of the metatarsophalangeal and interphalangeal joints, resulting in a characteristic "pencil-in-cup" deformity (arrowheads).

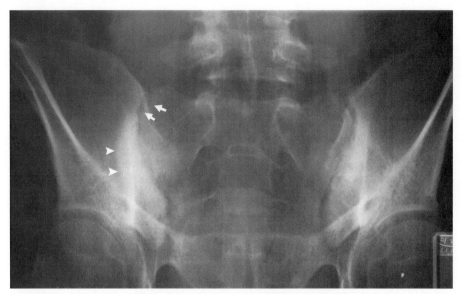

Figure 3.18   Ankylosing spondylitis

This radiograph demonstrates early changes of ankylosing spondylitis, including widening of the sacroiliac joints, diffuse subchondral sclerosis (arrowheads), and erosive changes characterized by irregularity of the cortical margin (arrows).

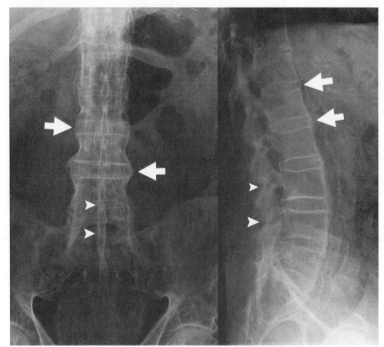

**Figure 3.19
Ankylosing spondylitis**

This radiograph demonstrates findings of advanced ankylosing spondylitis with thin vertical syndesmophytes at each disc space, resulting in fusion of the vertebral bodies and giving a "bamboo spine" appearance (arrows). A continuous line is seen in the middle of the lumbar spine on the AP radiograph, representing fusion of the spinous processes (arrowheads).

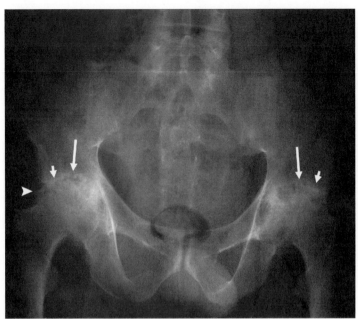

Figure 3.20
Ankylosing spondylitis, pelvis

This radiograph shows complete fusion of the sacroiliac joints, demonstrated by complete loss of the cartilage space and evidence of trabecular bone smoothly bridging the joint. Erosive and productive changes at the hips are also seen, including severe cartilage space narrowing, subchondral sclerosis (short arrows), erosions (long arrows), and osteophytes (arrowheads).

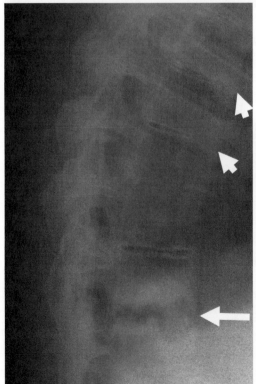

Figure 3.21   Ankylosing spondylitis

This lateral radiograph of the thoracic spine demonstrates thin anterior syndesmophytes at the anterior margins of the disc spaces (short arrows), except at T10-T11. At this level, there is widening, sclerosis, and irregularity due to a fracture through the disc space and formation of a pseudarthrosis (long arrow).

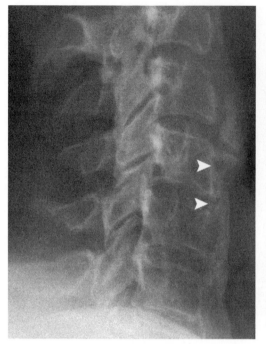

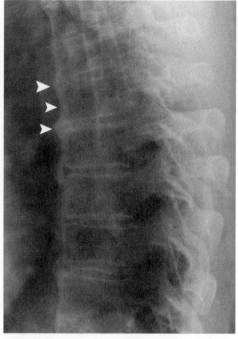

**Figure 3.22   Diffuse Idiopathic Skeletal
                Hyperostosis (DISH)**

This lateral radiograph of the cervical spine demonstrates
massively enlarged flowing osteophytes anterior to the
anterior margin of the vertebral bodies and bridging across
the disc spaces (arrowheads).

Figure 3.23   DISH

This lateral thoracic spine radiograph demonstrates
characteristic flowing anterior osteophytes bridging the
disc spaces and continuing anterior to the vertebral
bodies (arrowheads).

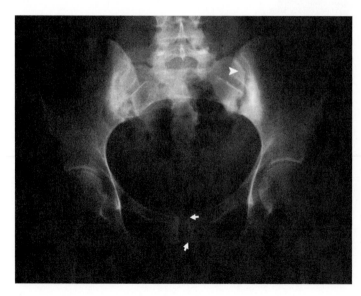

Figure 3.24   Reiter's disease

This AP radiograph of the pelvis
demonstrates asymmetric bilateral
sacroiliitis, with greater involvement
on the left demonstrated by increased
joint space widening on the left
(arrowheads). Pubic symphysitis with
erosions (arrows) is also noted.

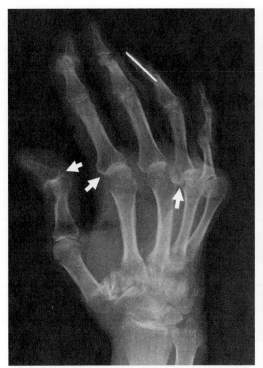
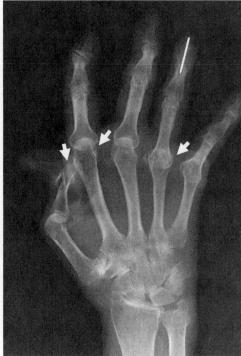

Figure 3.25   SLE

(A) PA and (B) oblique radiographs of the hand demonstrating severe subluxation at the second through fifth metacarpophalangeal joints and first interphalangeal joint (arrows). The subluxation results from ligamentous laxity and is the dominant finding in systemic lupus erythematosus.

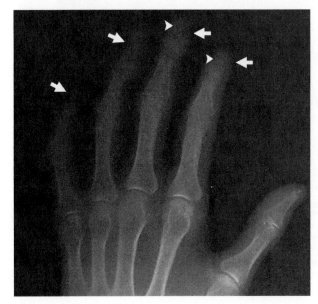

Figure 3.26   Scleroderma

This PA radiograph of both hands demonstrates distal tapering of the soft tissues of the digits (arrows) with acro-osteolysis at the distal tufts of the second and third digits (arrowheads). Soft tissue calcifications are seen at both the thumbs distally.

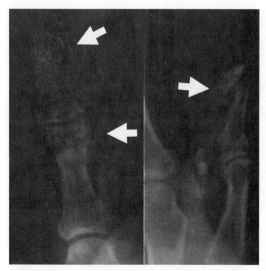 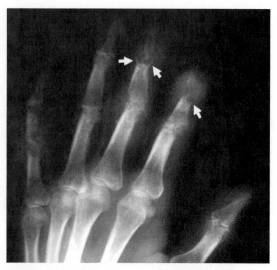

Figure 3.27   Scleroderma

These PA and lateral radiographs of the thumb demonstrate extensive soft tissue calcifications (arrows), as typically seen in scleroderma.

Figure 3.28   Gout

This PA radiograph of the fingers demonstrates multiple large well-defined para-articular erosions at the interphalangeal joints, with overhanging edges (arrows) and overlying tophi seen as dense soft tissue swelling.

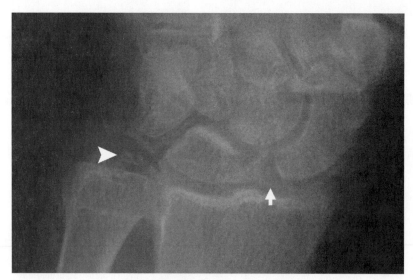

Figure 3.29   Pyrophosphate arthropathy

PA radiograph of the wrist, demonstrating characteristic findings of calcium pyrophosphate dihydrate crystal deposition disease (CPPD), including chondrocalcinosis of the triangular fibrocartilage complex (arrowhead), scapholunate ligament (arrow), as well as the hyaline cartilage of the scaphoid, lunate, and triquetrum. There is mild widening of the scapholunate interval.

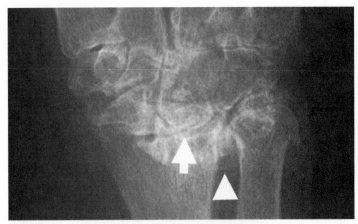

Figure 3.30
Pyrophosphate arthropathy

This PA radiograph of the wrist demonstrates advanced scapholunate collapse. There is scapholunate dissociation with dislocation of the lunate (arrowhead), articulation of the capitate with the radius (arrow), and proximal descent of the distal carpal row. Erosions and productive changes are seen at the metacarpophalangeal joints.

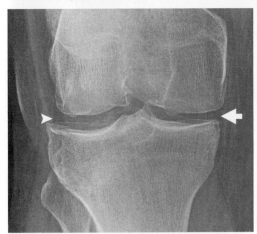

Figure 3.31   Pyrophosphate arthropathy

This AP radiograph of the knee demonstrates chondrocalcinosis of the hyaline cartilage of both the medial and lateral compartment (arrow on medial compartment) and chondrocalcinosis of the lateral meniscus (arrowhead).

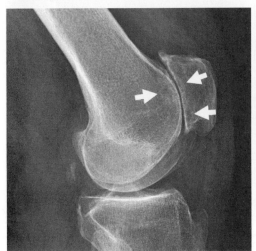

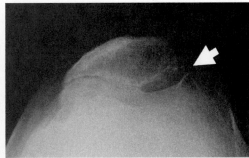

Figure 3.32   Pyrophosphate arthropathy

(A) Lateral and (B) sunrise knee radiographs demonstrate patellofemoral joint osteophytes and erosions (arrows). The dominant involvement in pyrophosphate arthropathy at the knee is at the patellofemoral joint.

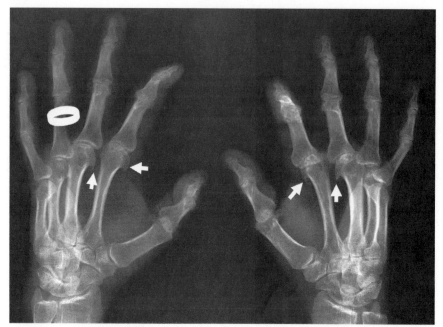

Figure 3.33   Hemochromatosis

On this PA view of the hand, large beaklike osteophytes (arrows) are seen at the second and third metacarpal heads, as well as cartilage space narrowing, erosions, and subchondral cystic changes. Chondrocalcinosis can be seen frequently, although it is not demonstrated in this patient.

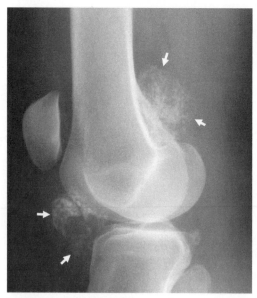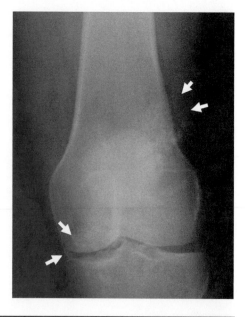

Figure 3.34   Synovial chondromatosis

(A) AP and (B) lateral radiographs of the knee demonstrate multiple large rounded ossified bodies within the joint space (arrows).

CHAPTER 4

Common Soft Tissue Pain Syndromes

Simon Helfgott, MD

OVERVIEW

The soft tissue pain syndromes are characterized by local or regional pain and discomfort that is often made worse by palpation of the adjacent soft tissue or movement of the nearby joint (**Table 4.1**). When they involve the soft tissues near a joint, they can be associated with decreased range of motion of that joint. The resultant lost of function can be significant. The diagnosis is based on the patient's history and physical examination. Imaging and laboratory testing, when indicated, may help to eliminate other diagnoses, but rarely confirm a soft tissue pain syndrome. Thus, many patients are either undiagnosed or misdiagnosed, leading to costly evaluations, including unnecessary imaging and costly therapeutics. This chapter will review some of the more common soft tissue pains syndromes, their clinical presentation, their physical examination findings, and their appropriate management.

Table 4.1 Clinical Features of Soft Tissue Pain Disorders

Presentation	Acute or subacute
Location	Focal usually asymmetrical pain though it may radiate to a wider area
Pain Description	Deep aching (tendonitis, bursitis) Paresthesiae (nerve entrapment)
Time of Discomfort	Often worst at night and with activities causing pressure over the area

CLASSIFICATION OF DISORDERS

Soft tissue pain can be categorized into a few major subsets:
- Tendonitis: common shoulder problems such as supraspinatus or bicipital tendonitis
- Bursitis: subacromial, olecranon, anserine, trochanteric
- Epicondylitis: medial and lateral
- Nerve entrapment syndromes: carpal or tarsal tunnel syndrome
- Regional pain syndromes: widespread pain in a region of the body (e.g., the upper back, chest wall, or an entire extremity)

- Generalized pain syndromes: chronic widespread pain syndrome, fibromyalgia, and whiplash injuries (**Table 4.2**)

Table 4.2   Generalized Soft Tissue Pain Syndromes

Fibromyalgia
Whiplash injuries (post motor vehicle crash)
Chronic Regional Pain Syndrome (CRPS)
Myofascial pain

PATHOPHYSIOLOGY

The pathophysiology of soft tissue pain syndromes is poorly understood. Because tissue biopsy is rarely, if ever, indicated, no good clinicopathologic correlations are available for most of these conditions, with the exception of carpal tunnel syndrome. In this disorder, the histopathology of excised soft tissue demonstrates scarring and fibrosis sometimes associated with an inflammatory infiltrate surrounding an entrapped median nerve. However, in most other disorders the findings may be minimal; for example, some patients with recurrent shoulder pain may have some thinning of the tendon sheaths with sparse inflammatory cell infiltrates and occasional fibrosis.

The bursae are synovial-lined sacs that help to facilitate joint motion by providing lubricated tissue for gliding. Generally, bursae are of two types: subcutaneous and deep. The subcutaneous bursae permit the movement of skin overlying the bursae. The deep bursae separate different tendon compartments or are present between tendons and bone. Generally, bursae contain trace amounts of acellular synovial fluid for optimal lubrication.

The causes of chronic widespread pain syndrome, fibromyalgia, and regional pain syndromes remain unknown. The common feature to all these conditions is that the musculoskeletal areas that are symptomatic are not the actual pain-generating sites. Mounting evidence suggests that these disorders are caused by alterations in the body's processing of pain signals either at the level of the brain or the spinal cord.

PRESENTATION

The onset of soft tissue pain disorders can be acute or insidious. An antecedent history of excessive physical activity may have predisposed the patient to injury. Generally, patients will complain of the onset of a localized discomfort, and they can usually point to an area of maximal pain. The pain is described as throbbing, dull, and aching. Pain symptoms are usually worse during periods of inactivity and rest. For example, patients will often note the pain at night, and it may awaken them from sleep or prevent them from getting to sleep. A patient with trochanteric or subacromial bursitis may notice the pain mostly when lying on the affected side. Similarly, nerve entrapment pain, such as that from carpal tunnel syndrome, is often worse at night. Presumably, with sleep, the patient is unable to maintain a proper wrist position that would prevent irritation to the nerve. These nocturnal exacerbations are in contrast to the situation in patients with an inflammatory arthritis such as rheumatoid arthritis (RA). In those patients, nighttime pain is uncommon and, when present, suggests the development of a soft tissue pain disorder superimposed on their RA.

PATIENT DEMOGRAPHICS AND COMMON PRESENTATIONS

Soft tissue pain syndromes can affect patients of either sex with about equal frequency and at any age. The exception would be fibromyalgia, which is seen far more frequently in females. Some specific types of soft tissue pain syndromes are seen in certain populations.

Patients with shoulder pain due to supraspinadus tendonitis, subacromial bursitis, or bicipital tendonitis often present with an antecedent history of excessive use. In younger patients, this might relate to athletic activities that require repeated external rotation and abduction at the shoulder. Sports such as baseball and tennis can precipitate these episodes. In older patients, these shoulder problems are often associated with structural changes that have occurred at the shoulder due to aging. For example, the presence of an osteophyte near the rotator cuff mechanism may result in a partial tear or fraying of the cuff tendons. These patients often present with pain and a marked limitation of mobility. This is in contrast to patients with shoulder bursitis or tendonitis, where pain limits active motion but passive range of motion can generally be achieved.

Medial and lateral epicondylitis are the most common causes of elbow pain. In longstanding cases, the pain can radiate distally toward the wrist and hand, mimicking other conditions, such as carpal tunnel syndrome. It is often precipitated by repetitive hand squeezing and gripping maneuvers. The most common causes include excessive use of the computer mouse or work tools, such as hammers or screwdrivers, and sports that require a firm grip on the equipment, such as tennis or golf.

Carpal tunnel syndrome may be associated with repetitive overuse of the hands, although the data are conflicting. Other causes include marked obesity; pregnancy; inflammatory arthritis, such as RA; hypothyroidism; diabetes mellitus; and, rarely, amyloidosis. These systemic disorders should be considered when patients present with bilateral symptoms.

Trochanteric bursitis is usually seen in two groups of patients. The first group includes obese patients whose weight continually stresses the soft tissues surrounding the hip joint. The second group includes patients who have rapidly increased their level of physical and athletic activities, resulting in excessive stresses around the hip and thigh.

The most common causes of soft tissue pain around the knee are anserine bursitis and patellofemoral dysfunction. The anserine bursa sits inferior and medial to the knee and can be distinguished from pain due to osteoarthritis by the presence of exquisite tenderness reproduced by palpation over the bursa. These patients are older and usually have some degree of underlying medial knee joint cartilage loss consistent with osteoarthritis. Patellofemoral dysfunction results in pain being felt over the knee when attempting to initiate activities that require knee flexion and extension. This is often present in younger woman and presents with pain primarily when going down more than up stairways, and the patients often have a small non-inflammatory joint effusion and mild quadriceps atrophy.

Pain around the ankle and foot may include Achilles tendonitis as well as tendonitis affecting the extensor tendons (more often than the flexor tendons) of the foot. Tendonitis around the ankle and foot is often related to increased levels of physical activity, or it may be related to underlying altered foot biomechanics, such as pes planus (flat foot). Achilles tendonitis tends to occur in younger athletic individuals; a change in footwear may predispose certain patients to its development. A history of recent quinolone antibiotic use can predispose some patients to tendon rupture, especially the Achilles tendons.

SPECIFIC SOFT TISSUE PAIN DISORDERS

Shoulder Pain

Shoulder pain is a common disorder. It may be caused by problems within the shoulder joints (i.e., the glenohumural, acromioclavicular, or sternoclavicular joints) or from one of the periarticular structures, such as the rotator cuff or bicipital tendons; the shoulder joint capsule; or the subacromial bursa. Less commonly, the pain is referred to the shoulder from a nerve impingement in the cervical spine or brachial plexus or at the thoracic outlet. In some cases, the pain may originate from a lesion in the diaphragm or the right upper quadrant of the abdomen, such as in acute cholecystitis. Pain originating from the glenohumeral joint or the rotator cuff is generally felt just a few centimeters distal to the shoulder joint margin over the deltoid muscle area. Pain that is felt above the shoulder may not be emanating from the shoulder and suggests either a cervical radiculopathy or a soft tissue injury above the shoulder with radiation of the pain toward the shoulder. Pain that is felt behind the shoulder joint is most likely due to subscapularis tendon injuries or referred pain from cervical spine disease.

Bilateral shoulder pain may be a feature of a systemic disorder, such as polymyalgia rheumatica or RA. Osteoarthritis of the glenohumeral joint is very uncommon except in cases where there was an antecedent shoulder joint injury or prior metabolic damage to the cartilage, as seen in chondrocalcinosis.

Patients may describe a history of insidious onset of pain. Those who have an abrupt onset of pain during activity may be describing a partial tear of an affected tendon (e.g., a rotator cuff tear). These patients will often present with marked inability to raise the arm. Why is tendonitis so common in the shoulder region? This is because during shoulder abduction the rotator cuff and long bicep tendons are subjected to impingement at the greater tuberosity of the humerus and the coracoacromial arch. With excessive or frequent repetitive overhead activities, tissue injury results in tears of the rotator cuff as well as tendonitis within the cuff mechanism. A viable rotator cuff is required for both abduction and external rotation of the shoulder as well as stabilizing the glenohumeral joint and preventing the superior migration of the humeral head. Thus, an injured or damaged rotator cuff may be unable to prevent some degree of superior migration of the humeral head. This results in further damage to the rotator cuff and to the long biceps tendon (which sits on the humeral head), which are now being squeezed by the changing architecture of the joint. With time and recurrent injury, osteophytes may form over the inferior surface of the acromioclavicular joint, and this will intensify the degree of impingement of the rotator cuff and the biceps tendon. Thus, the spectrum of these chronic impingement syndromes can range from episodes of mild tendonitis of the rotator cuff to the development of rotator cuff or long head of the bicep tendon tears. Since the subacrominal bursa is adjacent to the rotator cuff, many of these cases are also associated with a subacrominal bursitis.

Table 4.3   Common Soft Tissue Disorders by Site

Shoulder	Rotator cuff tendonitis Bicipital tendonitis Subacromial bursitis
Elbow	Medial or lateral epicondylitis Olecranon bursitis
Wrist	DeQuervain's tenosynovitis Flexor tenosynovitis Dupuytren's contracture Carpal tunnel syndrome
Hip/Pelvis	Trochanteric bursitis Ischial bursitis Iliopsoas bursitis
Knee	Medial (no name) bursitis Anserine bursitis Pre- and infrapatellar bursitis Patellofemoral dysfunction
Ankle and Foot	Achilles tendonitis Retrocalcaneal bursitis Plantar fasciitis Morton's neuroma

Some patients may have a sudden onset of explosive, exquisitely painful shoulder pain with marked difficulty with any range of motion. Such patients are extremely uncomfortable and are very reluctant to comply with a physical examination of the shoulder.

Radiographs of the affected shoulder demonstrate calcification within the rotator cuff tendon or subacromial bursa. These calcified deposits often disappear following resolution of the episode.

The physical examination of the shoulder should begin with inspection for evidence of muscle wasting or bony hypertrophy over the acromioclavicular joint. Such findings suggest a longstanding problem. Shoulder fullness (suggesting effusion) is unusual and not easily visualized, because a shoulder joint effusion would be deep within the tissues and is diagnosed through imaging such as magnetic resonance imaging (MRI) or shoulder ultrasound.

Shoulder range of motion and function is assessed by having patients place their arm by their side and slowly raise it laterally to assess the range of shoulder abduction. The first 30 to 40 degrees of abduction are controlled by the deltoid muscle. Beyond 40 degrees, abduction is performed using the rotator cuff mechanism. Patients with rotator cuff-related tendonitis or impingement syndromes will have a definite loss of motion and a description of pain with abduction beyond 40 degrees. The patients continue this motion against the resistance of the examiner's hand, which is placed on the patients' elbow while applying downward pressure. The patients' ability to continue abduction against resistance is noted; if the patients complain of pain, the diagnosis of a rotator cuff-related injury (either tendonitis or tear or both) is made. A rotator cuff tear can be distinguished from tendonitis if the patients are unable to actively abduct the arm beyond 40 degrees but can passively move the arm through this arc of motion without pain.

Patients who have a subacromial bursitis may note local tenderness on palpation of the subacromial bursa that sits at the top of the humerus just below the glenoid arch. Patients with a bicipital tendonitis often describe pain that is felt more anteriorly over the top part of the humerus, corresponding to the bicep tendon insertion area. However, note that many patients may have features of each of these conditions because the affected areas are in close proximity to one another.

Other related structures also affect the shoulder joint's range of motion, in addition to the glenohumeral joint, the rotator cuff and the acromioclavicular joint. Limitation of sternoclavicular motion (arthritis or trauma) or scapulothoracic motion (isolated muscle dystrophies or isolated palsy of the long thoracic nerve) may limit the normal range of motion of the true shoulder joint.

Elbow Pain

The most common causes of elbow pain are medial and lateral epicondylitis. Although initially described as "tennis elbow," lateral epicondylitis is more commonly seen with activities such as excessive computer mouse use or repeated gripping of work tools, such as screwdrivers and hammers. These activities all require repeated, frequent use of the hand flexor tendons. Although initially considered a form of tendonitis with suspected inflammation at the tendon bone insertion interface, it is now considered by some to be a cumulative trauma overuse disorder, with repetitive mechanical overloading of the common extensor tendon, particularly involving the portion derived from the extensor carpi radialis brevis tendon. In some histopathologic specimens of excised epicondylar tissue, there is evidence of fibroblastic hyperplasia and disorganized collagen bundles.

The pain often is insidious and sometimes bilateral, although it usually involves the dominant arm. The pain is generally localized to the lateral epicondyle, but over time it may extend both distally toward the wrist and proximally upward toward the shoulder. It is exacerbated by any squeezing activities of the hands, such as those involved in holding a pen or gripping or lifting objects. Such pain can be confirmed by having the patient try to squeeze an object such as a cup; this will often elicit the pain. Palpation over the lateral epicondylar area usually provokes intense pain and discomfort. However, the elbow range of motions, such flexion and extension, as well as pronation and supination, are maintained. One way to distinguish epicondylitis from a true elbow joint arthritis is to assess pronation and supination range of motion. In patients with elbow joint synovitis, these motions are reduced; there is no effect on these motions with either type of epicondylitis.

Medial epicondylitis is less common than the lateral form. Although known as "golfer's elbow," the condition is more common in patients who are at risk for lateral epicondylitis as well. Typically, the patient has an antecedent history of cumulative repetitive strain of the common flexor muscle of the forearm, provoking pain and tenderness at the medial epicondylar region. The pain may radiate proximally and distally as well. The diagnosis is confirmed by noting pain over the medial epicondyle with either palpation or by the simultaneous forced full extension of the elbow and the wrist.

Olecranon Bursitis

The olecranon bursitis sits below the tip of the elbow and can become swollen and sometimes painful due to a number of conditions. These include trauma, inflammation (e.g., due to RA or gout), or sepsis. Gouty bursitis and infection can both be associated with similar findings, such as increased warmth, swelling, and redness along with pain, and thus it is generally necessary to aspirate the bursa for synovial fluid analysis, including cell count, gram stain, and culture of the joint fluid. Septic olecranon bursitis is usually the result of direct inoculation of bacteria via a skin abrasion and can occur in otherwise healthy individuals engaged in physical work that results in frequent trauma to the elbows. The most common pathogen is *Staphylococcus aureus*. Traumatic bursitis can occur with recurrent or incidental trauma to the elbow. Patients often present because of swelling that may be only minimally painful. The diagnosis is confirmed by joint aspiration demonstrating hemorrhagic joint fluid with few white blood cells, no bacteria, or crystals being present.

Wrist and Hand Pain

Perhaps the most common soft tissue disorder involving the wrist and hand is carpal tunnel syndrome. This disorder is caused by entrapment of the median nerve within the carpal tunnel. It is characterized by painful paresthesiae and sensory loss in a median nerve distribution. Generally, this involves the thumb, the second digit, and half of the third digit. More advanced cases may have loss of motor power in the median distribution in the hands as well as atrophy of the thenar muscles. Patients generally present with a history of nocturnal pain in the median nerve distribution. Percussion of the median nerve at the flexor retinaculum just radial to the palmaris longus tendon at the distal wrist crease (Tinel's sign) will produce paresthesiae in the median nerve distribution. Phalen's sign is the development of paresthesiae following sustained palmar flexion of the wrist for 20 to 30 seconds. The severity of the entrapment and the need for surgical decompression can be assessed by electromyography.

Flexor tendon entrapment syndromes of the digits can occur in patients without a history of inflammatory arthritis or diabetes. Most cases are idiopathic, although patients with diabetes and RA may be at increased risk for this condition. Patients present with triggering symptoms involving a digit, especially following periods of inactivity such as arising in the morning. They often must use their other hand to help "unlock" the affected digit. A nodular thickening of the tendon is often present at the site of maximum tenderness, which is generally in a part of the flexor tendon just proximal to the metacarpophalangeal (MCP) joint of the affected digit. The histopathology of the lesion consists of hypertrophy and fibrocartilaginous metaplasia of the ligamentous layer of the tendon sheath, resulting in stenosis of the tendon sheath canal and mechanical entrapment of the tendon.

De Quervain's Tenosynovitis

De Quervain's tenosynovitis is a disorder affecting the common tendon sheath of the abductor pollicis longus and extensor pollicis brevis tendons. It is characterized by pain over the radial aspect of the wrist that is aggravated by movements of the thumb during pinching, grasping, and lifting activities. It is a tendon entrapment syndrome that results in the thickening of the extensor retinaculum that covers the first compartment of the wrist and leads to a tendon entrapment. Palpation of the affected tendon sheath re-creates pain and exquisite tenderness. Using Finkelstein's test, the patient makes a fist with the fingers wrapped around the thumb and then is instructed to flex the thumb in the ulnar direction. This reproduces the pain and confirms the diagnosis.

Dupuytren's Contracture

Dupuytren's contracture is caused by a nodular thickening and contracture of the palmar fascia, leading to marked flexion deformities of the fingers. It most commonly affects the ring finger, but it can involve any of the others. It may start in the ring finger flexor tendons and then continue to involve all the others. It can involve one or both hands. With the tendon scarring that develops, there is a gradual development of a flexion deformity of the fingers at the level of the MCP joints and an inability to fully extend the digits. The histopathology demonstrates fibrous nodules, proliferating fibrosis, and myofibrosis in the palmer fascia.

Pelvis and Hip Pain

There are three major bursae around the pelvis and hip region: the ischiogluteal, iliopsoas, and trochanteric bursae. The trochanteric bursae comprise three bursae, with the largest and most important one clinically separating the fibers of the gluteus maximus muscle from the greater trochanter. The other two bursae lie between the greater trochanter and the gluteus medius and greater trochanter, respectively.

Trochanteric bursitis presents with a deep aching pain over the lateral aspect of the upper thigh that is made worse by walking but also noted to be painful at night when the patient is laying on the affected side. The diagnosis is confirmed by obtaining a history of pain both at rest and with activity but in the presence of a normal range of motion of the affected hip joint. Additionally, there is pain with palpation over the trochanteric bursa. The pain may radiate distally but rarely beyond the knee. Risk factors include overuse activities such as excessive walking or running and improper footwear. The differential diagnosis of trochanteric bursitis includes lumbar radiculopathy involving the L1 and L2 nerve roots and the uncommon meralgia paresthetica, a syndrome characterized by entrapment of the lateral cutaneous nerve of the thigh, resulting in discomfort in the same region. Unlike bursitis, these patients tend to have more dysesthesiae symptoms than pain.

Ischiogluteal bursitis presents with pain over the ischial tuberosity. Previously known as "weaver's bottom," it is caused by repeated leg flexion and extension in the sitting position or prolonged sitting on hard surfaces. Diagnosis is confirmed by eliciting tenderness on palpation over the ischial tuberosity with the patient lying supine and the hip and knee flexed.

The iliopsoas bursa lies over the anterior surface of the hip joint. In most cases of iliopsoas bursitis, communication between the hip joint and the bursa appears to occur, and this may allow for a transfer of excess synovial fluid from one region to the other. The predisposing factors for excess synovial fluid include osteoarthritis, RA, and septic arthritis. The typical presentation consists of the onset of painful swelling in the inguinal area. When there is adjacent femoral vein or nerve compression, the resulting pain and or swelling may involve the entire leg.

Knee Pain

The three major bursae around the knee can become inflamed or infected, resulting in pain. The three major bursae around the knee are the prepatellar, infrapatellar, and anserine bursa.

The prepatellar bursa lies anterior to the patella and can become infected in patients who frequently kneel. Presumably, skin breakdown occurs, resulting in bacterial infection, most commonly *S. aureus*. It is characterized by superficial swelling over the dorsum of the patella with surrounding redness and erythema. Rarely, the patient may have systemic complaints such as fever and chills.

The infrapatellar bursa lies between the upper portion of the tibial tuberosity and the prepatellar ligament. It is separated from the knee joint synovium by a fat pad. Similar to prepatellar bursitis, excessive kneeling may cause skin breakdown in the region, resulting in infection. Some patients may have noninfectious inflammatory swelling of the bursa.

The anserine bursa lies under and adjacent to the pes anserinus, which is the insertion of the thigh adductor complex consisting of the sartorius, gracilis, and semitendinosus muscles. This region is about 5 centimeters below the medial aspect of the knee joint space. Pain in this area is often referred to *anserine bursitis*. Predisposing factors include underlying osteoarthritis of the medial knee compartment and excessive physical stress to the knee. Patients will often describe nocturnal pain that awakens them, and this can help to distinguish this condition from osteoarthritis, which is rarely painful at night except if there is end-stage osteoarthritis in the knee that would require total knee replacement. Women more commonly develop anserine bursitis, perhaps due, in part, to having a broader pelvic area, leading to greater tension caused by greater angulation of the knee adductors. Obesity is another risk factor.

A "no name bursa" is found over the medial joint margin of the knee. Some clinicians believe that this bursa, when inflamed, can lead to intense medial knee pain. However, medial knee pain can also be due to osteoarthritis, trauma, and ligamentous injury.

The iliotibial band, which connects the ilium with the lateral tibia, can become painful due to the repetitive flexion and extension with running, resulting in iliotibial band syndrome. On examination, the patient experiences tenderness over the lateral femoral condyle approximately 2 centimeters above the joint line, with pain on weight bearing when the knee is flexed at about 40 degrees. Correction of the problem with foot orthotics can be helpful.

Formerly known as chrondromalacia patella, patellofemoral pain syndrome refers to poorly localized anterior knee pain that is often made worse when the patient initiates activities such as getting up from a seated position. Pain felt over the entire knee, and it is often made worse by forced flexion or extension of the affected knee. It is thought to result from anatomic abnormalities resulting in abnormal angulation of the patellar surface so that it becomes misaligned with the rest of the knee. Other theories include repetitive microtrauma to the patellar surface. This condition is more commonly seen in women, but it can occur in patients of either sex and at all ages. Radiographs of the knee are often unremarkable. Intensive physical therapy to enhance the strength of the medial aspect of the quadriceps mechanism is often helpful in alleviating symptoms.

Foot Pain

The most common soft tissue disorders around the ankle and feet include Achilles tendonitis, retrocalcaneal bursitis, and plantar fasciitis. They share a common causation, because these conditions are typically seen in patients who have a pes planus deformity resulting in altered foot biomechanics and excessive stress over other parts of the bone and soft tissue. The Achilles tendon can become inflamed and in rare cases can tear. Risk factors for tear include recent use of quinolone antibiotics. Achilles tendonitis can also be the presenting manifestation of a spondyloarthropathy.

Retrocalcaneal bursitis may be confused with Achilles tendonitis because the bursa lies between the tendon and a fat pad adjacent to the talus. It can be caused by repetitive trauma, poor footwear, RA, and spondyloarthropathy.

Plantar fascia is a common condition thought to be due to repetitive microtrauma at the attachment site of the plantar fascia to the calcaneus, resulting in injury and inflammation. The patient experiences localized pain over the heel with weight-bearing activities and is worst with the initiation of walking activities. Although the vast majority of patients with this condition do not have an underlying arthropathy, in younger individuals it might be the initial presentation of a spondyloarthropathy. A careful history and musculoskeletal exam can help identify these patients.

Tarsal tunnel syndrome refers to the compression of the posterior tibial nerve as it courses through the canal adjacent to the tarsal bone. It is similar to carpal tunnel syndrome, with patients presenting with sensory dysesthesiae involving the plantar aspect of the foot. Nocturnal symptoms are worse and often awaken the patient. Percussion of the flexor retinaculum reproduces the symptoms. The patient may experience reduced vibratory sensation and decreased two-point discrimination over the planter aspect of the foot and toes. Diagnosis can be confirmed by nerve conduction studies documenting a delay in the nerve conduction of the posterior tibial nerve across the ankle.

Morton's neuroma is a condition that presents with paresthesiae or dysesthesiae in the interdigital web spaces, particularly between the third and fourth interspaces. The pain is increased by weight-bearing activities or by tight-fitting footwear. The patient experiences tenderness, and a clicking sensation is noted on simultaneous palpation of the web space while squeezing the patient's metatarsal bones with the other hand (Mulder's sign). The diagnosis can be confirmed by injection of a local anesthetic into the interspace, which should immediately, though temporarily, relieve symptoms.

ESTABLISHING THE DIAGNOSIS OF A SOFT TISSUE PAIN DISORDER

It is essential to take an accurate history and perform a thorough physical examination to rule out other causes that may mimic soft tissue pain syndromes. For example, radicular pain due to cervical or lumbar spine nerve entrapment can mimic some of the conditions described in this chapter. These patients usually describe a wider area of pain and generally lack specific focal areas of tenderness on palpation.

Another area of potential confusion, especially in the older patient, is the radiographic finding of osteoarthritis in adjacent joints. Sometimes these arthritic changes are ascribed as underlying cause for the patient's pain syndrome. However, it is important to recall that soft tissue pain has some unique characteristics that help to distinguish it from pain due to osteoarthritis. These include the finding of intense pain on palpation of the affected area along with the history of pain that is worse with rest and at night. Generally, osteoarthritis pain follows a reverse pattern, with pain improved with rest and sleep and made worse with activity. Palpation of an osteoarthritic joint does not generally exacerbate the pain to the same degree as is seen in soft tissue pain disorders.

Systemic diseases that sometimes need to be considered include polymyalgia rheumatica (in patients older than age 50 with persistent shoulder and hip girdle region discomfort), occult hypothyroidism, and, very rarely, vitamin D deficiency.

Ancillary Studies

For most soft tissue pain disorders, laboratory investigation should be minimal. When appropriate, a complete blood count (CBC), erythrocyte sedimentation rate (ESR), and C-reactive protein (CRP) might be useful. If there is a question of an underlying infectious process, an aspiration procedure should be considered.

Imaging of the affected area can be helpful in some situations. For example, in patients with an acute severe pain, fracture should be ruled out, especially if there is an antecedent history of trauma. If a calcific tendonitis is being considered, plain radiographs can confirm the diagnosis. In the case of periarticular knee pain thought to be due to bursitis, radiographs can assess the underlying cartilage loss and help exclude other mimics such as avascular necrosis or a nondisplaced stress fracture.

THERAPY

Treatment for most soft tissue disorders begins with patient education. For example, in overuse syndromes it is necessary for the patient to understand the underlying mechanism that predisposes one to the development of the pain syndrome and to be familiar with the measures to be taken to avoid these repetitive stresses in the future. Referral to physical therapy for stretching and exercise programs can be useful. Therapeutic modalities such as ultrasound provide a heat energy that can penetrate into the deep soft tissues. For carpal tunnel syndrome, proper wrist splinting, especially at night, can provide some symptom relief (see **Table 4.4**).

Table 4.4   Therapeutic Options

Physical Therapy	Stretching Massage Electrical Stimulation Ultrasound Heat /Ice
Occupational Therapy	Splinting Joint immobilization
Medications	NSAIDs Acetaminophen Tramadol Mild narcotic analgesics Topical lidocaine Capsaicin cremes Intralesional corticosteroids

As mentioned earlier, an aspiration procedure should be seriously considered if infection is a diagnostic concern. Before injecting soft tissues, one must be certain that an underlying infection is not the cause of the problem. Injection of a corticosteroid preparation combined with lidocaine can provide symptomatic relief. For example, the combination of 20 to 40 mg of methylprednisolone along with 1 to 2 mL of 2% lidocaine can be injected into a bursa or near painful tendon structures to provide symptomatic relief. Generally, these injections can be performed at the bedside or in the office without assistive radiology guidance. Data suggest that patient outcomes following nonguided injections are equal to those administered with radiographic assistance.

Nonsteroidal anti-inflammatory drugs (NSAIDs) can provide some modest pain relief. Other analgesics, such as acetaminophen or tramadol, can be useful. Narcotic analgesics should be avoided except for those circumstances requiring short-term management of severe pain. Systemic corticosteroids are not indicated for any of the soft tissue pain disorders.

For patients whose symptoms persist despite the various therapeutic approaches, the possibility should be considered that there is an underlying structural causation for their pain. At this point, if imaging has not yet been performed it may be useful to assess the area radiographically.

Patients who have more widespread and persistent achiness may have an underlying disorder such as fibromyalgia causing the persistence of symptoms.

◇◇◇◇◇◇◇◇◇◇◇◇◇◇◇◇◇◇◇◇◇◇

SUGGESTED READINGS

Andres BM, Murrell GA. Treatment of tendinopathy: What works, what does not, and what is on the horizon. *Clin Orthop Relat Res.* 2008;466(7):1539–1554.

Barr KP. Review of upper and lower extremity musculoskeletal pain problems. *Phys Med Rehabil Clin N Am.* 2007;18(4):747–760.

Bennett R. Myofascial pain syndromes and their evaluation. *Best Pract Res Clin Rheumato.* 2007;21(3):427–445.

Burbank KM, Stevenson JH, Czarnecki GR, Dorfman J. Chronic shoulder pain: part I. Evaluation and diagnosis. *Am Fam Physician.* 2008;77(4):453–460.

Riley, G. Tendinopathy—from basic science to treatment. *Nat Clin Prac Rheumatol.* 2008;4:82–89.

Sharma P, Maffulli N. Biology of tendon injury: healing, modeling, and remodeling. *J Musculoskelet Neuronal Interact.* 2006;6(2):181–190.

CHAPTER 5

Back and Neck Pain

Simon Helfgott, MD

OVERVIEW

Most adults will experience at least one episode of low back pain or neck pain during their lifetime, yet these conditions remain a diagnostic and therapeutic challenge to many practitioners. Spine pain is subjective, and often few objective findings are identified during the physical examination and diagnostic evaluation of the patient.

Psychosocial and economic issues, such as litigation, workers' compensation claims, and depression, may have an impact on the management of the patient and the treatment outcome. Instead of performing an exhaustive search for the precise cause of spine pain, it is often more productive to address three questions:

- Is a systemic disease causing the pain?
- Are there neurologic findings requiring surgical evaluation?
- Are there any psychosocial factors that may adversely affect the pain?

This chapter provides a review of low back pain and neck pain.

BACK PAIN

Epidemiology

Low back pain is seen most frequently in patients between the ages of 20 and 40, but it is more severe in when it occurs in older patients. The sex distribution is equal. Approximately 2 to 8% of patients with low back pain develop chronic disabling pain. Risk factors include heavy lifting, twisting movements, and bodily vibrations (e.g., motor vehicle crashes), obesity, and poor conditioning.

Pathogenesis

Idiopathic Low Back Pain

Low back pain may emanate from spinal structures, including the nerve roots, facet joints, disks, vertebral bodies, and adjacent ligaments and soft tissues. However, in the majority of cases of isolated low back pain without neurologic deficits the origin of the pain cannot be discerned. These patients may be categorized as having an idiopathic low back pain. Other terms used to denote this entity include *low back strain* or *sprain* and *lumbago*.

Disk-Related Low Back Pain

The avascular intervertebral disks are complex anatomic structures that provide motion, neural element protection, and shock absorption in a highly efficient manner. The process of disk degeneration is thought to occur because of the disruption of the normal diffusion of oxygen, nutrients, and waste products through the avascular disk. This results in the development of annular tears, dehydration of the nucleus, and fissure development in the vertebral endplate cartilage. Over time, subchondral sclerosis of the endplates occurs. All of these changes alter the spinal biomechanics and may induce further structural changes, including cartilage degradation and osteophyte formation at the level of the facet joints.

Spinal Stenosis

Progressive narrowing of the neural foramina can result in the development of spinal stenosis. This may be caused by a combination of bony overgrowth (e.g., osteophyte formation, Paget's disease), disk protrusion or herniation, or congenital anomalies, such as shortened vertebral pedicles. Neural impingement is worsened by activities such as walking, and claudication-like symptoms usually require the patient to slow down or to stop and rest. Forward flexion of the spine may also relieve the pressure, and patients often acquire a forward flexed posture and learn to lean on objects (e.g., shopping carts) for symptom relief.

Tumor/Infection

A hallmark feature of back pain due to tumor or infection is the patient's description of an unremitting pain incompletely relieved by rest or lying down. When nerve roots or the cauda equina are impinged by mass lesions, the clinical features may resemble sciatica or the cauda equina syndrome. Infiltration of the vertebral bodies by a space-expanding lesion can result in fracture. Intervertebral disk space infiltration can cause focal or radiating pain

Diagnostic Evaluation

History

The majority of patients with low back pain suffer from the idiopathic form (i.e., a presumed strain or sprain that will likely improve with time). These patients complain of low back discomfort that does not radiate. A smaller percentage of patients have radicular symptoms with pain down either or both legs, sometimes with and sometimes without accompanying low back pain.

　　　Although neoplasms and infections probably account for less than 1% of all back pain, it is crucial that the history should focus on ruling out worrisome symptoms that may suggest these diagnoses. Factors that may increase the risk of neoplasms and infections include the patient's age (>50 years), a history of cancer, unexplained weight loss, fever, injection-drug use, chronic infection, unremitting pain, nighttime pain, and a lack of response to prior therapy.

Key elements of the history should also include the characterization of the pain and determining whether there are symptoms suggesting neurologic involvement (see **Table 5.1**). These symptoms include leg pain with walking (pseudoclaudication), numbness, or paresthesia. Sciatica due to disk herniation typically worsens with coughing, sneezing, or with the Valsalva maneuver.

Table 5.1 Clinical Aspect of Low Back Pain

Type	Findings	Neurologic*	Causation
Idiopathic	Non radiating pain + soft tissues tenderness	No	Injury, overuse
Disk degeneration	Focal back pain may be aggravated by extension	No	Aging
Sciatica	Shooting pain radiating along the leg	Yes	Nerve root impingement by disk and/or osteophytes
Neurogeneic claudication	Buttock/thigh/leg pain with activity. Improves with rest or forward flexion	Yes	Spinal stenosis due to multi disk protrusions; congenital narrowing of the spinal canals
Spondyloarthropathy	Back stiffness worsened by inactivity	Uncommon	HLA-B27-related conditions
Fracture	Focal, unrelenting pain	No	Direct trauma, osteoporosis
Tumor, Infection	Focal, unrelenting pain + systemic features	Occasionally	Metastatic disease, primary tumors, infectious lesions

* Neurologic findings include loss or attenuation of deep tendon reflexes; altered sensation following a dermatome distribution; reduction in strength of distal lower extremities.

Bowel or bladder dysfunction (e.g., retention with overflow incontinence), perianal anesthesia, leg weakness, and sciatica may be features of cauda equina compression. Patients suspected of having this syndrome require urgent surgical evaluation.

Finally, prolonged back pain may be influenced by psychosocial issues, including depression, somatization, and legal issues related to compensation claims.

Physical Examination

Most patients will describe pain in the lower back, buttocks, or legs; palpation of these areas is generally not helpful in establishing the diagnosis. For example, vertebral tenderness has sensitivity for infection (diskitis) but lacks specificity for other diagnoses. Similarly, the presence of limited spinal mobility is a nonspecific finding and can be observed in a wide array of conditions that cause back pain.

The straight-leg-raising (SLR) test is performed with the patient supine and the uninvolved knee bent to 45 degrees and resting on the table. The examiner's hand holds the leg straight, cups the heel with the other hand, and gradually raises the leg. When there is a disk herniation irritating the nerve roots, the SLR will further stretch these roots and pain will radiate below the ipsilateral knee, not merely in the back and hamstring muscles. A positive test occurs with an elevation of the leg of less than 60 degrees. Ipsilateral pain is sensitive but not specific for a herniated disk, whereas pain down the opposite leg (crossed SLR) is highly specific but lacks sensitivity. The value of the SLR decreases with advancing age.

The neurologic examination should focus on the ankle and knee reflexes, ankle and big toe dorsiflexion strength, and the distribution of sensory complaints (**Table 5.2**).

Table 5.2   Disk Levels Nerve Roots Findings

Disk Levels	Nerve Roots	Findings
L2-4	L3/L4	Reduced knee jerk/ reduced strength in quads and iliopsoas strength, dysesthesiae in thigh and knee
L4-5	L5	Reduced strength in the extensor hallucis longus tendon. Dysesthesiae in 1st toe and medial part of the foot
L5-S1	S1	Reduced ankle jerk and toe flexors, dysesthesiae in the 5th toe and the lateral foot
Any central herniation	S2-S4	Dysesthesiae in the perineum bowel/bladder dysfunction

Imaging Studies

Lumbar spine radiography is generally not helpful in the evaluation of patients with acute low back pain because the radiographic findings are generally age-related changes. Exceptions may include the finding of vertebral compression fractures or structural anomalies such as spondylolisthesis or scoliosis. Although radiographic features of sacroiliitis may be evident only years after the onset of disease, earlier changes such as straightening of the lumbar spine, vertebral body squaring, and syndesmophyte formation may be seen earlier. Lumbar radiography is not highly sensitive for detecting early cancer or infection.

Current guidelines recommend plain radiography in patients with fever, unexplained weight loss, neurologic deficits, injection-drug abuse, or age older than 50, although structural abnormalities, such as spondylolisthesis and scoliosis, can be easily detected.

Computed tomography (CT) and magnetic resonance imaging (MRI) have similar accuracy in detecting herniated disks and spinal stenosis. MRI studies have revealed the presence of herniated disks in 22 to 40% and bulging disks in 24 to 81% of asymptomatic adults. Thus, MRI studies need to be interpreted cautiously. These studies should be reserved for patients for whom there is a strong clinical suspicion of underlying infection, cancer, or persistent neurologic deficit. MRI or CT imaging may be helpful in planning for epidural steroid injections or to ascertain whether surgical referral is appropriate.

Clinical Course

Although some studies have suggested that pain resolves within a few weeks of onset in the vast majority of patients, symptoms may recur in many patients with idiopathic low back pain. Similarly, most patients with disk herniations will improve, although a small subset—perhaps 10% of patients—may require a surgical referral because of ongoing pain or worsening neurologic deficits. Patients with spinal stenosis may experience remissions and relapses over time. Back pain due to an axial spondyloarthropathy will generally improve with the initiation of an aggressive exercise program coupled with the use of nonsteroidal anti-inflammatory drugs (NSAIDs) or, in more severe cases, the use of anti-TNF-alpha blocking drugs. Pain caused by vertebral compression fractures will usually improve within 4 to 6 weeks.

Treatment

Idiopathic Low Back Pain

Most patients with idiopathic low back pain should be encouraged to return to normal activities as soon as possible. Prolonged or excessive bed rest is not recommended. If necessary, work modifications should be implemented to allow the patient a gradual return to full activities. Pain relief can be provided with regular dosing of NSAIDs prescribed for the duration of symptoms. Muscle relaxants such as cyclobenzaprine may be helpful for short-term relief of nighttime discomfort. The use of narcotic analgesics generally should be avoided. Spinal chiropractic manipulation, physical therapy, and acupuncture may provide limited benefit.

Disk Herniation

Many patients will slowly improve within the first 4 to 6 weeks. They should be treated similar to patients with idiopathic low back pain; however, given the more intense nature of the pain, they may require more potent analgesia for pain relief. Mild narcotic analgesics and gabapentin may be helpful for treating radicular symptoms. If radicular pain persists, and there is a good neuroanatomic correlation between imaging findings and the patient's examination findings, targeted epidural steroid injections may offer symptomatic relief.

The indications for surgical referral include the development of a cauda equina syndrome, a worsening neurologic deficit, or a persistent motor deficit.

Spinal Stenosis

No clear-cut effective treatment is available for spinal stenosis. There is a variable response and limited data regarding the benefits of physical therapy, NSAIDs, analgesics, and epidural steroid injections. MRI studies have identified spinal stenosis in one-fifth of asymptomatic individuals older than age 60, thus referral to surgery should be limited to those patients with clinical features of stenosis, such as neurogenic claudication or lower extremity weakness and pain. Patients experiencing a progressive decline in functional status (e.g., walking shorter distances, developing a greater need for analgesics) or unremitting leg pain may need to consider surgical decompression. Surgery may provide better pain relief and functional recovery than nonsurgical therapies, at least for a few years. However, a relapse of symptoms can occur years later.

Conclusion

With time, the majority of patients with low back pain will improve. The clinician needs to identify those patients who demonstrate symptoms or signs suggestive of a more serious process. Careful attention should be paid to the neurologic exam. Imaging studies generally can be avoided or delayed for several weeks and utilized judiciously. A rational approach to pain management should be employed. Using this stepwise approach may obviate the need for excessive testing and the use of questionable remedies.

NECK PAIN

Disorders affecting the cervical spine can be divided into conditions that predominantly cause neck pain and those that often cause extremity pain and/or neurologic dysfunction. Neck pain can be caused by cervical strain, disc disruption syndrome/discogenic pain, cervical facet-joint mediated pain, "whiplash" syndrome, and myofascial pain. Disorders that predominantly cause extremity symptoms and/or neurologic dysfunction include cervical radiculopathy and cervical spondylitic myelopathy.

The cervical spine is composed of seven vertebrae. The articulation between the occiput and the first cervical vertebra (the atlanto-occipital joint) allows for approximately one-third of flexion and extension and one-half of lateral bending of the neck. The articulation between the first and second cervical vertebrae (the atlantoaxial joint) allows for 50% of rotational range of motion. The articulations between the second and seventh cervical vertebrae allow for approximately two-thirds of flexion and extension, 50% of rotation, and 50% of lateral bending. The role of the cervical and trapezius muscles is to support and provide movement and alignment for the head and neck and to protect the spinal cord and spinal nerves when the spinal column is under mechanical stress.

Pain emanating from the cervical spine is generally felt around the neck and above the shoulders. When there is neural impingement due to disk herniation, the symptoms of pain and dysesthesiae and weakness are observed in the upper extremity. This is analogous to what is seen in patients with sciatica and disk herniation in the lower back. The pain is generally associated with some degree of cervical and paracervical muscle spasm; movement of the neck, particularly lateral flexion, may worsen symptoms. The finding of intense, painful dysesthesiae radiating down the neck into the spine, known as L'hermitte's sign, is a worrisome finding. It may be seen in patients with cervical spinal cord pathology due to demyelination or in cases of cervical myelopathy.

Because the spinal cord passes through the cervical spine, the clinician needs to ascertain whether there is evidence for spinal cord compression. Findings indicating compression include intense pain; numbness and dysesthesiae down the arms and sometimes the legs; clumsy hand movements; motor weakness, such as worsening or sluggish gait; and bowel or bladder dysfunction.

Patients with erosive forms of rheumatoid and juvenile rheumatoid arthritis have a greater risk of atlantoaxial subluxation (C1-C2) and these patients need to be carefully screened for features of neurologic impingement.

The Physical Examination

A detailed upper extremity neurologic examination should be performed in all patients with neck pain. This should include muscle strength testing, assessment of deep tendon reflexes, and a sensory exam. A negative neurologic examination indicates a low likelihood of root compression; positive findings, however, are not specific for root compression.

The majority of patients presenting with a sensory radiculopathy have a good prognosis and respond to conservative measures. In contrast, patients with sensorimotor involvement (with or without spinal cord compression) have a less predictable prognosis; they are more likely to have more dramatic degrees of disk herniation, are at higher risk for nerve damage, and are more likely to require surgical intervention.

In general, assessment of strength, reflexes, and sensory examination, in combination with patient symptoms, can target a specific root lesion:

- C4 radiculopathy may affect the levator scapular and trapezius muscles, resulting in weakness in shoulder elevation. There is no reliable associated reflex.

- C5 radiculopathy is associated with weakness of the rhomboid, deltoid, bicep, and infraspinatus muscles. Patients may have weakness of shoulder abduction and external rotation. The bicep reflex may be diminished.
- C5-C6 paracentral and/or foramenal herniation or foramenal stenosis at C5-C6 affects the C6 nerve root and produces pain at the shoulder tip and trapezius, with radiation to the anterior upper arm, radial forearm, and thumb and sensory impairment in these areas. Weakness involves flexion at the elbow or shoulder external rotation. The bicep or brachioradialis reflex may be diminished.
- C6-C7 paracentral and/or foramenal herniation or foramenal stenosis at C6-C7 affects the C7 nerve root and produces pain at the shoulder blade, pectoral area, and medial axilla, with radiation to the posterolateral upper arm, dorsal elbow and forearm, index and medial digits or all of the fingers, and sensory impairment in these areas. Weakness involves the elbow extensors and forearm pronators. There may be a diminished tricep reflex.
- C7-T1 paracentral and/or foramenal herniation or foramenal stenosis at C7-T1 causes C8 radiculopathy. Clinically, patients present with symptoms similar to an ulnar or median motor neuropathy and can have weakness of finger abductors and grip strength; they may also have findings suggesting median motor neuropathy. No reliable reflex test is available.

Causes of Neck Pain Syndromes

Cervical Strain

Cervical strain is a nonspecific diagnosis used to describe an injury to the cervical paraspinal muscles and ligaments with associated spasm of the cervical and upper back muscles. This diagnosis implies a normal neurologic exam.

Cervical strain may result from the physical stresses of everyday life, including poor posture and sleeping habits. Typically, symptoms are experienced as pain, stiffness, and tightness in the upper back or shoulder and may last for several weeks.

Cervical Spondylosis

Degenerative changes in the cervical spine are apparent on radiographs of many adults older than age 30. The term *cervical spondylosis* encompasses soft tissue and disc damage and degenerative bony lesions. The abnormalities include a sequential change in the intervertebral discs, with osteophyte formation along the vertebral bodies, and changes in the facet joints and laminal arches. However, the correlation between the degree of radiographic change and the presence or severity of pain is poor.

Cervical Discogenic Pain

The degenerative process that occurs in the intervertebral disc is associated with an inability to effectively distribute pressures between the disc, vertebral endplates, and facet joints. Cervical discogenic pain refers to derangement in the architecture of the disc that results in mechanical neck pain with or without features of inflammation. Axial pain is more severe than extremity pain. When present, extremity pain is thought to result from somatic referral rather than spinal nerve root impingement. Symptoms are often exacerbated when the neck is held in one position for prolonged periods. There is often associated muscle tightness and spasms.

Physical examination should demonstrate axial neck discomfort with range of motion, a decreased range of motion, and a benign neurologic examination.

Cervical Facet Syndrome

Historically, patients often have a history of trauma with an abrupt flexion-extension type injury or an occupation that leads to repeatedly positioning the neck in extension. Pain is often midline or offset slightly to one side. Symptoms can be somatically referred to the shoulders, periscapular region, occiput, or proximal limb. As with cervical discogenic pain, axial symptoms are greater than extremity symptoms.

Whiplash Injury

The cervical "whiplash" syndrome is caused by a traumatic event with an abrupt flexion/extension movement to the cervical spine. Symptoms of whiplash include severe pain, spasm, loss of range of motion in the neck, and occipital headache. Pain can be persistent with little identifiable abnormality seen on MRI, CT, radiograph, or bone scan imaging. The injury is common but remains poorly understood.

Cervical Myofascial Pain

Regional pain with associated trigger points and pressure sensitivity has been called *myofascial pain*. It can be a nonspecific manifestation of any pathologic condition that causes pain from the neck to the shoulder and should not be considered a defining diagnosis. Associated features may include a heightened soft tissue pain sensitivity, depression, and insomnia.

Causes of Extremity Pain and/or Neurologic Deficit

Cervical Spondylotic Myelopathy

Cervical spondylotic myelopathy is defined by degenerative changes narrowing the spinal canal, resulting in cervical spinal cord injury or dysfunction. Cervical spondylotic myelopathy can result from an extradural mass, as seen with bony osteophyte formation, herniated nucleus pulposus, or ossification of the posterior longitudinal ligaments, cervical spondylolisthesis, or congenital narrowing of the spinal canal. Patients may present with various neurologic complaints: weakness, coordination impairment, gait disturbance, bowel or bladder retention or incontinence, and sexual dysfunction.

Spinal cord compression due to spondylotic change tends to occur in the lower cervical spine; degenerative changes are more severe and more common between C5 and T1 and the spinal cord is enlarged between C4 and T2.

The differential diagnosis for cervical spondylotic myelopathy includes multiple sclerosis, syringomyelia, tumor, epidural abscess, and amyotrophic lateral sclerosis. Because optimal neurologic recovery depends on early surgical decompression, distinguishing cervical spondylotic myelopathy from other causes of neck pain is critical.

Cervical Radiculopathy

Cervical radiculopathy refers to dysfunction of the spinal nerve root that may manifest with pain, weakness, reflex changes, or sensory changes. Degenerative changes in the spine are overwhelmingly the most common cause, accounting for up to 90% of cases. Other possible causes include cervical foramenal stenosis, cervical herniated disc, herpes zoster and diabetic polyradiculopathy.

Nonspinal Causes of Neck Pain

Thoracic Outlet Syndrome

The thoracic outlet syndrome can present as neck and shoulder pain with referred pain to the upper extremities and variable neurovascular signs and symptoms. The triad of numbness, weakness, and a sensation of swelling of the upper limbs is strongly suggestive of thoracic outlet syndrome. Examination may demonstrate a positive Roos sign (repetitive and vigorous handgrip while the arms are abducted overhead) or a positive Adson's test (diminution of the radial pulse when the arm is abducted, extended backward, the head is turned ipsilaterally, and the patient inspires).

Herpes Zoster

Herpes zoster (shingles) may present with unilateral radicular symptoms without neurologic findings. The rash may not appear for several days after the onset of pain.

Diabetic Neuropathy

Diabetes mellitus can be associated with various neuropathic pain syndromes. Cervical and thoracic polyradiculopathy, plexopathy, and peripheral entrapments can be associated with neck, thoracic, scapular, and extremity pain and/or weakness.

Other Causes

Although the majority of neck pain complaints are related to musculoskeletal causes, numerous other conditions can present with a constellation of symptoms that include neck pain. The diagnosis of these conditions is usually evident from accompanying symptoms (e.g., fever, neck stiffness, diffuse joint pain):

- Malignancy: tumors involving the cervical spinal column
- Vascular: vertebral artery or carotid artery dissection
- Cardiovascular: angina and myocardial infarction
- Infection: pharyngeal abscess, meningitis, subdiaphragmatic abscess, herpes zoster
- Visceral: esophageal obstruction, biliary disease, apical lung tumor
- Referred shoulder pain: impingement, rotator cuff tear
- Rheumatologic: polymyalgia rheumatica, fibromyalgia

◇◇◇◇◇◇◇◇◇◇◇◇◇◇◇◇◇◇◇◇◇◇

SUGGESTED READINGS

Andersson GBJ. Epidemiologic features of chronic low-back pain. *Lancet.* 1999;354:581–585.

Deyo RA, Weinstein JN. Low back pain. *N Engl J Med.* 2001;344:363–370.

Deyo RA, Rainville J, Kent DL. What can the history and physical examination tell us about low back pain? *JAMA.* 1992;268:760–765.

Gibson JNA, Grant IC, Waddell G. The Cochrane review of surgery for lumbar disc prolapse and degenerative lumbar spondylosis. *Spine.* 1999;24:1820–1832.

CHAPTER 6

Osteoarthritis

Yvonne C. Lee, MD

OVERVIEW

Osteoarthritis is a common musculoskeletal disorder that stems from cartilage degradation at joint sites, leading to significant pain and disability. Overall, clinical osteoarthritis, defined by symptoms and physical examination findings, affects 12.1% of the U.S. population, ages 25 to 74 years. This percentage corresponds to approximately 26.9 million adults in the United States. The prevalence of osteoarthritis increases with age and is more common among women than men.[1]

Osteoarthritis may be defined radiographically or symptomatically. Radiographic osteoarthritis is assessed by joint space narrowing, sclerosis, and the presence of osteophytes, which are bony outgrowths at the joint margins. Radiographic osteoarthritis is more common than symptomatic osteoarthritis, and the prevalence varies depending on the affected joints. Among adults 26 years of age or older, the prevalence of radiographic osteoarthritis ranges from 14% at the knees to 27% at the hands, whereas the prevalence of symptomatic osteoarthritis ranges from 5% at the knees to 7% at the hands (**Table 6.1**).[1]

Table 6.1   Prevalence of Osteoarthritis in Population-based Studies[1]

Site	Study	Age (years)	Radiographic Osteoarthritis (%)	Symptomatic Osteoarthritis (%)
Hands	Framingham[2]	≥26	27	7
Knees	Framingham[3]	≥26	14	5
	Johnston County[4]	≥45	28	16
Hips	Johnston County[5]	≥45	27	9

PATHOGENESIS

Despite the high prevalence of osteoarthritis, its pathogenesis is not well understood. Articular cartilage degradation occurs early in the disease process, affecting joints in a focal, nonuniform pattern. Cartilage degradation is followed by bony remodeling, resulting in thickening of subchondral bone and osteophyte formation. Local synovial inflammation may occur in conjunction with damage to the cartilage and bone (**Table 6.2**).

Table 6.2   Tissues Affected in Osteoarthritis

Tissue	Findings
Cartilage	Cartilage loss
Bone	Osteophytes, subchondral bone sclerosis
Synovium	Focal inflammation

RISK FACTORS

Osteoarthritis may be primary (idiopathic) or secondary to a known cause. Risk factors for primary osteoarthritis include age, female sex, obesity, and trauma (**Table 6.3**). The risk of primary hip and knee osteoarthritis is increased by sports and recreational activities, particularly activities that predispose to injury, and occupational activities such as jumping, lifting, and climbing.[6] The association between mechanical factors and primary hand osteoarthritis is not well defined, but there is likely a balance between use (which is protective) and overuse (which is damaging).[7]

Secondary osteoarthritis occurs after joint and, in particular, meniscal surgery and in patients with inflammatory joint disease (e.g., chondrocalcinosis, gout, rheumatoid arthritis, and septic arthritis), metabolic disease (e.g., acromegaly, hemochromatosis, hyperparathyroidism, and Paget's disease), and hypermobility syndromes (e.g., Ehlers-Danlos syndrome) (Table 6.3).

Table 6.3   Risk Factors for Primary and Secondary Osteoarthritis[8,9]

Primary Osteoarthritis	Secondary Osteoarthritis
Age	Joint surgery (e.g., meniscal surgery)
Female sex	Crystal arthritis (e.g., chondrocalcinosis and gout)
Obesity	Inflammatory arthritis (e.g., rheumatoid arthritis, septic arthritis)
High bone mass	Acromegaly
Occupations requiring physical labor (e.g., lifting heavy objects, standing for long periods of time)	Hemochromatosis
Weight-bearing sports (for competitive athletes)	Hyperparathyroidism
History of trauma/injury	Paget's disease
Genetic predisposition/family history	Hypermobility syndromes (e.g., Ehlers-Danlos syndrome)

DIFFERENTIAL DIAGNOSIS

The differential diagnosis depends on the site of involvement. It may include inflammatory and crystalline arthritis (e.g., rheumatoid arthritis, seronegative spondyloarthropathies, gout, and chondrocalcinosis), septic arthritis, bursitis, tendonitis, meniscal/ligamentous tears, and iliotibial band syndrome.

DIAGNOSIS

The American College of Rheumatology (ACR) has published criteria for the clinical and radiographic classification of hand, knee, and hip osteoarthritis.[10–12] Although originally developed to classify patients for clinical trials, these criteria have also been used to guide the diagnosis of osteoarthritis (**Table 6.4**).

Table 6.4   ACR Classification Criteria for Osteoarthritis of the Hands, Knees, and Hips

SITE	CLASSIFICATION CRITERIA
Hands[10]	Hand pain, aching or stiffness and three of the four following criteria: 1. Hard tissue enlargement of two or more of ten selected joints 2. Hard tissue enlargement of two or more DIP joints 3. Fewer than three swollen MCP joints 4. Deformity of at least one of ten selected joints
Knees[11]	Knee pain, osteophytes, and at least one of the three following criteria:* 1. Age older than 50 years 2. Stiffness less than 30 minutes 3. Crepitus
Hips[12]	Hip pain and at least two of the three following criteria: 1. Erythrocyte sedimentation rate (ESR) of less than 20 mm/hr 2. Radiographic femoral or acetabular osteophytes 3. Radiographic joint space narrowing

*Clinical and radiographic criteria for classification of osteoarthritis of the knees. The ACR has also published clinical criteria and clinical and laboratory criteria.

A comprehensive medical history should include assessment of the location and timing of pain as well as the presence of morning stiffness. Primary osteoarthritis tends to affect the distal interphalangeal (DIP), proximal interphalangeal (PIP), and carpometacarpal (CMC) joints of the hands, hips, knees, and cervical or lumbar spine. Individuals with osteoarthritis usually have increased pain with activity and decreased pain with rest. Morning stiffness tends to last less than 30 minutes. Night pain may indicate another etiology, such as inflammatory or crystalline arthritis, infection or tumor, or osteoarthritis severe enough to justify surgical intervention.

On physical examination, swelling and erythema should be noted and range of motion fully assessed. Individuals with hand osteoarthritis may have enlargements of the DIP and PIP joints, known as Heberden's and Bouchard's nodes. Squaring of the CMC joint may also be evident. In individuals with knee osteoarthritis, crepitus may be detected upon movement of the knee joint, and asymmetric narrowing of the medial and lateral compartments may lead to varus and valgus deformities, respectively. Individuals with osteoarthritis of the feet may present with bunions and hallux rigidus (immobility of the first metatarsophalangeal joint).

No blood tests are needed to diagnosis osteoarthritis, though physicians may want to check inflammatory markers if the history or examination suggests an inflammatory arthritis. Similarly, synovial fluid examination is not required unless an alternative diagnosis is suspected. When performed, synovial fluid analysis usually reveals white blood cell counts $\leq 2000/mm^3$.

Radiographs are helpful to confirm the diagnosis of osteoarthritis and exclude other causes. Characteristic radiograph findings include osteophytes, joint space narrowing, and sclerosis. For osteoarthritis of the knees and hips, standing films should be obtained, because they may reveal abnormalities that are not evident on non-weight-bearing films. Magnetic resonance imaging (MRI) may also be performed, but due to its high cost it should only be ordered when circumstances are concerning for alternative etiologies. Although radiographic studies provide important supplemental information, they should not be the sole criterion for diagnosis and treatment, because findings are inconsistently correlated with pain and function.[13,14]

TREATMENT

At present, no disease-modifying antiosteoarthritis drugs are available. The current treatment of osteoarthritis is focused on relieving pain and preventing disability. Most randomized, controlled trials have concentrated on individuals with knee osteoarthritis. Although findings from these studies have been extrapolated to apply to osteoarthritis at other sites, few studies have actually assessed the roles of pharmacologic and nonpharmacologic interventions in osteoarthritis at these sites (i.e., hips and hands).[15]

In 2000, the ACR published recommendations for the treatment of osteoarthritis of the hip and knee. These guidelines included both pharmacologic and nonpharmacologic interventions (**Figure 6.1**), as well as surgery for severe cases.[16]

Nonpharmacologic Treatments

Nonpharmacologic interventions, such as exercise and weight loss, are important components of osteoarthritis therapy. For individuals with knee osteoarthritis, quadriceps strengthening may decrease joint space narrowing.[17] Patient education and self-manage-

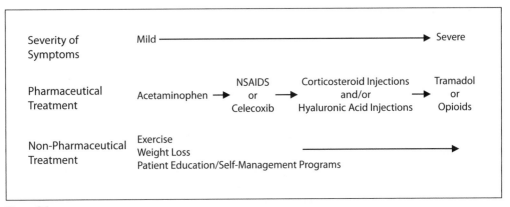

Figure 6.1

Multimodal therapy for osteoarthritis includes both pharmaceutical and nonpharmaceutical treatments.

ment programs are also recommended, although these programs likely have a greater impact on psychological outcomes than pain relief and physical function.[18] Recent studies have suggested that nonconventional therapies, such as acupuncture, may also be effective.[19,20]

Pharmacologic Treatments

Pharmacologic treatment includes acetaminophen, nonsteroidal anti-inflammatory drugs (NSAIDs), glucosamine chondroitin, corticosteroid injections, hyaluronic acid injections, tramadol, and opioid analgesics. Compared to placebo, both acetaminophen and NSAIDs relieve pain from hip and knee osteoarthritis, although the magnitude of relief is small.[21]

Gastrointestinal (GI) side effects are more common among those taking oral NSAIDs than those taking placebo or acetaminophen.[22] NSAIDs have also been associated with renal toxicity, so renal function should be monitored while patients are on chronic NSAID therapy. Alternatives to oral NSAIDs include topical NSAIDs, selective cyclooxygenase-2 (COX-2) inhibitors, and concurrent use of gastroprotective agents (i.e., proton pump inhibitor).[21]

Recent events (i.e., recall of rofecoxib) have highlighted the increased risk of cardiovascular events associated with COX-2 inhibitors. The risk of myocardial infarction is higher among patients taking COX-2 inhibitors compared to those taking placebo or naproxen. However, the risk of cardiovascular events associated with COX-2 inhibitors is comparable to the risk of cardiovascular events associated with other NSAIDs (excluding naproxen). Cardiovascular risk is dose-dependent; thus COX-2 inhibitors should be initiated at the lowest possible dose and optimally administered once daily (i.e., celecoxib 200 mg daily).[23]

If acetaminophen, NSAIDs, and COX-2 inhibitors are ineffective or contraindicated, intra-articular injections of corticosteroids and hyaluronic acid may be used for pain relief. Intra-articular injections of the hips should only be done with radiographic guidance. Botulinum toxin has also been employed for intra-articular injections.

Corticosteroid injections reduce pain during the first few weeks following injection, but there is little evidence for more prolonged effects. Injections are generally limited to once every 3 months. The long-term effects of repeated corticosteroid injections have not been well studied. Comparisons between corticosteroids suggest that triamcinalone hexacetonide may be more effective than betamethasone.[24]

Hyaluronic acid injections are most effective 5 to 13 weeks postinjection.[25] Data from head-to-head comparisons of hyaluronic acid products are limited,[25] although a recent meta-analysis suggests that hylan, a product consisting of cross-linked hyaluronic acid molecules, is associated with a higher risk of local adverse events than hyaluronic acids.[26] However, these medications have been approved as a "device," and double-blind placebo-controlled studies have not been performed comparing hyaluronate injections to other more traditional therapies.

For patients with severe pain, tramadol or opiate medication may be used. Tramadol is associated with small improvements in pain and function, but it is also associated with a two to three times higher risk for side effects. Common side effects include somnolence, dizziness, nausea, vomiting, constipation, and headache, and, ultimately, one out of eight individuals discontinue tramadol due to adverse effects.[27]

The role of nutraceuticals, such as glucosamine chondroitin, in the treatment of osteoarthritis is controversial. Initial studies suggested that glucosamine chondroitin was associated with moderate to large reductions in pain due to hip and knee osteoarthritis. However, many of these studies were small and of low quality. Furthermore, analyses indicated evidence of a bias towards the publication of positive studies (studies showing an association between glucosamine chondroitin and pain relief) compared to negative studies.[28] Recent large, randomized, controlled trials have not shown any benefit in the use of glucosamine chondroitin to treat pain from knee osteoarthritis.[29]

Surgery

Surgical interventions for osteoarthritis range from arthroscopic debridement to total joint replacement. Arthroscopic debridement is largely ineffective in reducing pain and improving function.[30] Total hip and total knee replacements, in contrast, are two of the most cost-effective interventions in health care.

Indications for total joint replacement include severe pain and/or functional impairment due to hip or knee osteoarthritis, despite pharmacologic and nonpharmacologic therapy. The optimal timing for surgery depends largely on the individual patient and his or her perception of pain, disability, and the risk/benefit ratio of surgery. Older age is not a contraindication for total joint replacement, but patients with significant comorbidities, including obesity, are more likely to have poor functional outcomes and adverse events.[31]

Pain scores improve substantially 3 to 6 months postsurgery. Significant improvements in physical function also occur. Ten years postsurgery, overall revision rates are 7% for total hip replacements and 10% for total knee replacements.[32]

Total recovery time for total joint replacement may take several months. With the help of physical therapists, patients are usually able to start walking within 1 day of surgery. Patients are usually discharged after 4 to 5 days in the hospital. At discharge, many patients are still unable to walk independently, requiring a walker, crutches, or a cane to aid ambulation. The majority of patients are discharged to inpatient rehabilitation facilities.[33]

In patients with medial compartment knee osteoarthritis, unicompartmental knee replacement is also effective in reducing pain and improving function, although prosthesis survival may be slightly lower than total knee replacement. For young patients with medial compartment knee osteoarthritis who wish to delay total knee replacement, high tibial osteotomy may also be an effective option.[34]

CONCLUSION

Osteoarthritis is the most common type of joint disease, frequently affecting joints such as the hands, knees, and hips. Risk factors include age, female sex, and obesity. The exact pathogenesis of osteoarthritis is not well understood, but it involves cartilage degradation, bony remodeling, and local synovial inflammation. Current therapies for osteoarthritis are targeted at symptomatic relief and include both pharmacologic and nonpharmacologic treatments. The ultimate intervention for hip and knee osteoarthritis is total joint replacement.

◇◇◇◇◇◇◇◇◇◇◇

REFERENCES

1. Lawrence RC, Felson DT, Helmick CG, Arnold LM, Choi H, Deyo RA, et al. Estimates of the prevalence of arthritis and other rheumatic conditions in the United States. Part II. *Arthritis Rheum* 2008;58(1):26–35.

2. Zhang Y, Niu J, Kelly-Hayes M, Chaisson CE, Aliabadi P, Felson DT. Prevalence of symptomatic hand osteoarthritis and its impact on functional status among the elderly: The Framingham Study. *Am J Epidemiol.* 2002;156(11):1021–1027.

3. Felson DT, Naimark A, Anderson J, Kazis L, Castelli W, Meenan RF. The prevalence of knee osteoarthritis in the elderly. The Framingham Osteoarthritis Study. *Arthritis Rheum.* 1987;30(8):914–918.

4. Jordan JM, Helmick CG, Renner JB, Luta G, Dragomir AD, Woodard J, et al. Prevalence of knee symptoms and radiographic and symptomatic knee osteoarthritis in African Americans and Caucasians: the Johnston County Osteoarthritis Project. *J Rheumatol.* 2007;34(1):172–180.

5. Helmick CG, Renner JB, Luta G, Dragomir AD, Kalsbeek WD, Abbate LM. Prevalence of hip pain, radiographic hip osteoarthritis (OA), severe radiographic hip OA, and symptomatic hip OA: The Johnston County Osteoarthritis Project. *Arthritis Rheum.* 2003;48(Suppl 9):S212.

6. Vignon E, Valat JP, Rossignol M, Avouac B, Rozenberg S, Thoumie P, et al. Osteoarthritis of the knee and hip and activity: a systematic international review and synthesis (OASIS). *Joint Bone Spine.* 2006;73(4):442–455.

7. Kloppenburg M. Hand osteoarthritis—an increasing need for treatment and rehabilitation. *Curr Opin Rheumatol.* 2007;19(2):179–183.

8. Felson DT. Clinical practice. Osteoarthritis of the knee. *N Engl J Med.* 2006;354(8):841–848.

9. Lane NE. Clinical practice. Osteoarthritis of the hip. *N Engl J Med.* 2007;357(14):1413–1421.

10. Altman R, Alarcon G, Appelrouth D, Bloch D, Borenstein D, Brandt K, et al. The American College of Rheumatology criteria for the classification and reporting of osteoarthritis of the hand. *Arthritis Rheum.* 1990;33(11):1601–1610.

11. Altman R, Asch E, Bloch D, Bole G, Borenstein D, Brandt K, et al. Development of criteria for the classification and reporting of osteoarthritis. Classification of osteoarthritis of the knee. Diagnostic and Therapeutic Criteria Committee of the American Rheumatism Association. *Arthritis Rheum.* 1986;29(8):1039–1049.

12. Altman R, Alarcon G, Appelrouth D, Bloch D, Borenstein D, Brandt K, et al. The American College of Rheumatology criteria for the classification and reporting of osteoarthritis of the hip. *Arthritis Rheum.* 1991;34(5):505–514.

13. Dahaghin S, Bierma-Zeinstra SM, Hazes JM, Koes BW. Clinical burden of radiographic hand osteoarthritis: a systematic appraisal. *Arthritis Rheum.* 2006;55(4):636–647.

14. Bedson J, Croft PR. The discordance between clinical and radiographic knee osteoarthritis: a systematic search and summary of the literature. *BMC Musculoskelet Disord.* 2008;9:116.

15. Lee YC, Shmerling RH. The benefit of nonpharmacologic therapy to treat symptomatic osteoarthritis. *Curr Rheumatol Rep.* 2008;10(1):5–10.

16. Recommendations for the medical management of osteoarthritis of the hip and knee: 2000 update. American College of Rheumatology Subcommittee on Osteoarthritis Guidelines. *Arthritis Rheum.* 2000;43(9):1905–1915.

17. Mikesky AE, Mazzuca SA, Brandt KD, Perkins SM, Damush T, Lane KA. Effects of strength training on the incidence and progression of knee osteoarthritis. *Arthritis Rheum.* 2006;55(5):690–699.

18. Devos-Comby L, Cronan T, Roesch SC. Do exercise and self-management interventions benefit patients with osteoarthritis of the knee? A metaanalytic review. *J Rheumatol.* 2006;33(4):744–756.

19. Manheimer E, Linde K, Lao L, Bouter LM, Berman BM. Meta-analysis: acupuncture for osteoarthritis of the knee. *Ann Intern Med.* 2007;146(12):868–877.

20. White A, Foster NE, Cummings M, Barlas P. Acupuncture treatment for chronic knee pain: a systematic review. *Rheumatology* (Oxford). 2007;46(3):384–390.

21. Zhang W, Moskowitz RW, Nuki G, Abramson S, Altman RD, Arden N, et al. OARSI recommendations for the management of hip and knee osteoarthritis, part I: critical appraisal of existing treatment guidelines and systematic review of current research evidence. *Osteoarthritis Cartilage.* 2007;15(9):981–1000.

22. Towheed TE, Maxwell L, Judd MG, Catton M, Hochberg MC, Wells G. Acetaminophen for osteoarthritis. *Cochrane Database Syst Rev.* 2006(1):CD004257.

23. Laine L, White WB, Rostom A, Hochberg M. COX-2 selective inhibitors in the treatment of osteoarthritis. *Semin Arthritis Rheum.* 2008;38(3):165–187.

24. Bellamy N, Campbell J, Robinson V, Gee T, Bourne R, Wells G. Intraarticular corticosteroid for treatment of osteoarthritis of the knee. *Cochrane Database Syst Rev.* 2006(2):CD005328.

25. Bellamy N, Campbell J, Robinson V, Gee T, Bourne R, Wells G. Viscosupplementation for the treatment of osteoarthritis of the knee. *Cochrane Database Syst Rev.* 2006(2):CD005321.

26. Reichenbach S, Blank S, Rutjes AW, Shang A, King EA, Dieppe PA, et al. Hylan versus hyaluronic acid for osteoarthritis of the knee: a systematic review and meta-analysis. *Arthritis Rheum.* 2007;57(8):1410–1418.

27. Cepeda MS, Camargo F, Zea C, Valencia L. Tramadol for osteoarthritis. *Cochrane Database Syst Rev.* 2006;3:CD005522.

28. McAlindon TE, LaValley MP, Gulin JP, Felson DT. Glucosamine and chondroitin for treatment of osteoarthritis: a systematic quality assessment and meta-analysis. *JAMA.* 2000;283(11):1469–1475.

29. Clegg DO, Reda DJ, Harris CL, Klein MA, O'Dell JR, Hooper MM, et al. Glucosamine, chondroitin sulfate, and the two in combination for painful knee osteoarthritis. *N Engl J Med.* 2006;354(8):795–808.

30. Laupattarakasem W, Laopaiboon M, Laupattarakasem P, Sumananont C. Arthroscopic debridement for knee osteoarthritis. *Cochrane Database Syst Rev.* 2008(1):CD005118.

31. Lubbeke A, Stern R, Garavaglia G, Zurcher L, Hoffmeyer P. Differences in outcomes of obese women and men undergoing primary total hip arthroplasty. *Arthritis Rheum.* 2007;57(2):327–334.

32. Lobo ED, Loghin C, Knadler MP, Quinlan T, Zhang L, Chappell J, et al. Pharmacokinetics of duloxetine in breast milk and plasma of healthy postpartum women. *Clin Pharmacokinet.* 2008;47(2):103–109.

33. de Pablo P, Losina E, Phillips CB, Fossel AH, Mahomed N, Lingard EA, et al. Determinants of discharge destination following elective total hip replacement. *Arthritis Rheum.* 2004;51(6):1009–1017.

34. Brouwer RW, Raaij van TM, Bierma-Zeinstra SM, Verhagen AP, Jakma TS, Verhaar JA. Osteotomy for treating knee osteoarthritis. *Cochrane Database Syst Rev.* 2007(3):CD004019.

CHAPTER 7

Rheumatoid and Inflammatory Arthritis

Derrick J. Todd, MD, PhD

OVERVIEW

Joint pains (arthralgias) are a common complaint among patients who seek medical care. Arthralgias often are related to benign or self-limited processes, but it is important for the evaluating physician to identify patients in whom arthralgias may signal a serious underlying medical condition. Inflammatory arthritides represent one class of musculoskeletal disorders that, if left unrecognized, can lead to chronic inflammation, joint destruction, and disability. Rarely, these diseases can have life-threatening consequences. This chapter will focus mainly upon rheumatoid arthritis (RA) and the various spondyloarthropathies (SPAs) in adults as the principal systemic inflammatory arthritides. It will address the epidemiology, clinical manifestations, diagnostic studies, and current treatment of these disorders.

In addition to RA and the SPAs, many other rheumatic diseases can have musculoskeletal involvement of varying degree (**Table 7.1**). These other conditions are the subjects of other chapters in this text and will not be addressed in detail here.

Much of this chapter will focus on how to make a diagnosis of RA or an SPA, which is done using a combination of clinical features, laboratory tests, and radiographic findings; no single test or imaging study can be used to diagnose these entities with absolute certainty. Classification criteria exist for various rheumatic disorders (e.g., **Tables 7.2** and **7.3**),[1,2] but these were designed primarily for the purposes of research studies to maximize diagnostic specificity. One should exercise caution when trying to use these classification criteria in a clinical care setting because there are occasional patients who present with atypical inflammatory arthritis and who do not meet specific classification criteria.

It is important that the primary care physician (PCP) and rheumatologist work closely together to ensure that patients with new-onset inflammatory arthropathies are readily identified and expeditiously referred to a rheumatologist for longitudinal care.[3] The goal of rheumatologic evaluation is to confirm the presence of a systemic rheumatic illness and initiate disease-appropriate treatment. Great strides have been made in recent years in the immunomodulatory treatment of RA and the SPAs. It is well established that early initiation of these so-called disease modifying antirheumatic drugs (DMARDs) retards the natural history of the following disorders: symptomatic arthritis, radiographic destruction, joint deformity, functional disability, morbidity, and possibly even mortality.

Table 7.1   Diseases Causing Inflammatory Arthritis

Inflammatory Joint Disorders	Other Inflammatory Processes
Rheumatoid arthritis	
Spondyloarthropathies: • Ankylosing spondylitis • Irritable bowel disease (IBD)-related arthropathy • Psoriatic arthritis • Reactive arthritis • Undifferentiated spondyloarthritis	Microcrystalline arthritis: • Monosodium urate (gout) • Calcium pyrophosphate dihydrate (pseudogout) • Basic calcium phosphate • Calcium oxalate
Other connective tissue diseases: • Polymyalgia rheumatica • Systemic lupus erythematosus • Sjogren's syndrome • Scleroderma • Dermatomyositis/polymyositis • Mixed connective tissue disease • Adult-onset Still's disease	Septic arthritis: • Suppurative bacterial arthritis • Lyme arthritis • Gonococcal arthritis • Mycobacterial arthritis • Whipple's disease • Fungal and parasitic arthritis • Viral arthritis • Postvaccine arthritis
Systemic vasculitis	Malignant arthritis
Sarcoid arthritis	Paraneoplastic arthritis
Acute rheumatic fever	
Undifferentiated arthritis	

Table 7.2   American College of Rheumatology Classification Criteria for Rheumatoid Arthritis[1]

Must meet four of the following seven criteria:

1. Morning stiffness >1 hour duration
2. Soft-tissue swelling or fluid in three or more joints simultaneously
3. Swelling involving wrists, metacarpophalangeal joints, or proximal interphalangeal joints
4. Symmetric arthritis
5. Rheumatoid nodules
6. Elevated rheumatoid factor
7. Radiographic erosion in the hand or wrist

Criteria 1–4 must be present for >6 weeks.

Criteria 2–4 must be witnessed by a physician.

Exclude other diagnoses as deemed appropriate.

Adapted from Arnett et al., 1988

Table 7.3   Modified New York Classification Criteria for Ankylosing Spondylitis[2]

Must meet one of three clinical criteria *and* have radiologic evidence of sacroiliitis.

CLINICAL CRITERIA	RADIOLOGIC EVIDENCE OF SACROILIITIS: UNILATERAL GRADE 3–4 OR BILATERAL GRADE 2–4
1. Low back pain for >3 months. Relieved by exercise, but not rest	Grade 0. Normal
2. Limited lumbar spine flexion/extension or lateral bending	Grade 1. Suspicious sacroiliitis
3. Reduced chest expansion	Grade 2. Minimal sacroiliitis: erosion or sclerosis without widening or narrowing of joint space
	Grade 3. Moderate sacroiliitis: erosion, sclerosis, widening, narrowing, or partial ankylosis
	Grade 4. Total ankylosis

Adapted from Goei The HS, et al.

EPIDEMIOLOGY AND ECONOMICS

RA and the SPAs afflict somewhat different patient populations, although overlap certainly exists (**Table 7.4**). RA is the most common inflammatory arthritis, affecting 0.5 to 1% of the U.S. adult population.[4] Women are disproportionately affected (3:1), as are patients of Northern European ancestry. Although patients can be of any age, RA most commonly presents at 20 to 60 years of age. Genetic and environmental factors both appear to convey risk for RA. HLA-DRB1*0401 and -DRB1*0404 are the strongest genetic risk factors for RA.[5] Cigarette smoking is also associated with RA.[6] The socioeconomic burden of inflammatory arthritis is tremendous and measures well into the billions of dollars.[7] Direct costs arise from office visits, medications, hospitalizations, and orthopedic procedures. Even greater are the indirect costs of chronic disability and lost labor in the workforce.

Depending on the disease context, the SPAs are subclassified into ankylosing spondylitis (AS), inflammatory bowel disease (IBD) arthropathy, psoriatic arthritis (PsA), postinfectious reactive arthritis (ReA), and undifferentiated SPA. These disease prevalences vary but are less common than RA (Table 7.4). Unlike RA, SPAs either have a predilection for men (AS and ReA) or show no gender predisposition (IBD arthropathy and PsA). Patients may have peripheral arthritis of the extremities, spinal arthritis, or both. Spinal arthritis is associated with the HLA-B27 antigen; it is present in up to 90% of patients with AS. However, HLA-B27 is not sufficient to cause disease, as it is present in up to 10% of individuals of North European ancestry.[8]

Table 7.4   Clinical and Demographic Features of Rheumatoid Arthritis and the Spondyloarthropathies

	RHEUMATOID ARTHRITIS	SPONDYLOARTHROPATHIES			
		ANKYLOSING SPONDYLITIS	IBD ARTHROPATHY	PSORIATIC ARTHRITIS	REACTIVE ARTHRITIS
Prevalence	0.5–1.0% overall	0.1–0.2% overall	Up to 20% of IBD	Up to 0.1% overall	Up to 0.05% overall
Gender	Female 3:1	Male 3:1	Male = Female	Male = Female	Male ≥ Female*
Race	Any	Any (white)	Any (white)	Any (white)	Any (white)
Age	Any (often 20–60 years)	Younger than 40 years	Any age	Any (35–50 years)	Any (20–40 years)
Dominant arthritis	Peripheral	Spinal	Peripheral or spinal	Peripheral or spinal	Peripheral or spinal
Peripheral arthritis pattern	Symmetric polyarthritis of small and large joints Hands and wrists commonly involved Spares distal interphalangeal joint	Asymmetric oligoarthritis of large joints in lower extremities Enthesitis Dactylitis	AS pattern	Can be resemble either an AS or RA pattern, although may include distal interphalangeal joint	AS pattern
Spine arthritis pattern	Cervical spine only	Sacroiliitis Ascending spondylitis	AS pattern	Sacroiliitis Any level with "skip lesions"	PsA pattern

* Male predominance in urogenital ReA; equal distribution in enterogenic ReA.

CLINICAL FEATURES OF THE INFLAMMATORY ARTHRITIDES

Articular Manifestations

Joint inflammation (synovitis) is a common feature of RA and the various SPAs. Distinguishing features of these disorders are listed in Table 7.4. Synovitis is characterized clinically by erythema, warmth, and swelling of affected joints with synovial hyperplasia and joint effusions. Inflammatory symptoms tend to be worst in the morning and improve with activity (i.e., morning stiffness). In contrast, primarily mechanical joint disorders lack these inflammatory features (**Table 7.5**). Prolonged inflammatory joint disease can lead to cartilage destruction, structural deformity, ankylosis (joint fusion), and accelerated secondary osteoarthritis (OA), a common cause of disability and joint replacement surgery.

Table 7.5   Distinguishing Features of Inflammatory Versus Mechanical Arthritis

	INFLAMMATORY ARTHRITIS	MECHANICAL ARTHRITIS
Morning stiffness	Prolonged (>30 min)	Brief (<30 min)
Pattern over course of day	Improves	Worsens
Relationship to activity	Improves	Worsens
Joint findings	Red, warm, swollen joints Effusions Synovial thickening Tenosynovitis	Acute injury: red, warm, and swollen joints Chronic degeneration: bulky boney deformity
Classically spared joints	RA: lumbosacral spine	Primary OA: shoulders, elbows, wrists, metacarpophalangeal joints, ankles*
Synovial fluid (arthrocentesis)	>1500 white blood cells/mm³	<1500 white blood cells/mm³
Radiologic Findings	Osteopenia Erosions Cartilage loss	Sclerosis Osteophytes Cartilage loss

*Osteoarthritis at these atypical joints should suggest secondary causes of OA, including prior inflammatory arthritis, posttraumatic stress, endocrine disorders, etc.

RA tends to occur as a symmetric polyarthritis of the small and large joints of the extremities, almost always including the hands and wrists. Involvement of the feet is common as well, so careful foot examination should be part of any RA evaluation. Bursitis and tenosynovitis may also occur in RA and can lead to entrapment neuropathies such as carpal tunnel syndrome. Polyarticular features of RA are not absolute, however, and a small proportion of patients with RA may present with a persistent inflammatory monoarthritis that may or may not progress to polyarthritis.[9] RA spares the thoracolumbar spine, and cervical spine disease is discussed later.

Unlike RA, the SPAs have a propensity to affect the lumbar spine in addition to peripheral joints. Spinal arthritis often causes prolonged morning stiffness that improves with exercise. It typically starts in the lumbosacral area and progresses as an ascending spondylitis, but skip lesions can occur. If present in a young individual (younger than 40 years old), these symptoms should prompt a consideration of an SPA.[8] Peripheral joint disease in SPAs can resemble an RA-like pattern or it can exist as an asymmetric oligoarthritis primarily affecting the large joints of the lower extremities. Inflammation of a digit (dactylitis) and inflammation at the tendon-to-bone interface (enthesitis) are also features of the SPAs. Patients may also have costochondritis and reduced chest excursion that leads to restrictive lung disease.

Extra-Articular Disease

Patients with RA or SPAs may demonstrate various extra-articular manifestations of disease (**Table 7.6**). In both conditions, it is not uncommon for patients with uncontrolled inflammation to show systemic features of chronic illness: fatigue, fevers, night sweats, weight loss, anemia of chronic disease, and thrombocytosis. In patients with RA, other extra-articular features occur more commonly (but not exclusive) in seropositive patients who have detectable levels of rheumatoid factor or anti-cyclic citrullinated peptide (anti-CCP) antibodies (detailed below). Serious extra-articular manifestations (e.g., vasculitis) rarely occur in the setting of well-controlled disease, but conditions such as interstitial lung disease or nodular disease may occur despite treatment. In patients with SPAs, some of these features may be part of their disease association (e.g., psoriasis or IBD). Others, such as IgA nephropathy or aortitis, may occur in the setting of chronic uncontrolled inflammation.

Table 7.6   Extra-Articular Features of Rheumatoid Arthritis and the Spondyloarthropathies

ORGAN OR SYSTEM	RHEUMATOID ARTHRITIS	SPONDYLOARTHRITIDES
Systemic disease	Fever, weight loss, fatigue	Fever, weight loss, fatigue
Skin and mucous membranes	Rheumatoid nodules Cutaneous vasculitis	Psoriasis Pyoderma gangrenosum Keratoderma blenorrhagicum Circinate ballanitis
Lungs	Rheumatoid nodules Interstitial lung disease Bronchiolitis obliterans with organizing pneumonia (BOOP) Bronchiectasis Pleural effusions Pulmonary artery hypertension	Restricted chest excursion Apical pulmonary fibrosis
Cardiovascular system	Raynaud's syndrome Pericardial effusion Myocarditis Increased cardiovascular risk	Aortitis
Kidneys	Membranous glomerulonephritis Secondary amyloid	IgA nephropathy Secondary amyloid
Nervous system	Cervical myelopathy Entrapment neuropathies Peripheral nerve vasculitis	Cervical myelopathy Spinal stenosis

(continues)

Table 7.6   Extra-articular Features of Rheumatoid Arthritis and the Spondyloarthropathies

ORGAN OR SYSTEM	RHEUMATOID ARTHRITIS	SPONDYLOARTHRITIDES
Gastrointestinal tract	Transaminitis	Inflammatory bowel disease
Eyes	Keratoconjunctivitis Uveitis Episcleritis Scleritis Scleromalacia perforans Corneal ulceration	Uveitis
Mucous membranes	Aphthous ulcers Sicca	Aphthous ulcers Urethritis

Hematologic	Anemia
	Thrombocytosis
	Leukopenia
	Reactive lymphadenopathy
	Macrophage activation
	  syndrome (juvenile
	  rheumatoid arthritis)
	Felty's and LGL syndromes
	Increased lymphoma risk
		Anemia
		Thrombocytosis

Disease associations and overlap syndromes	Systemic lupus erythematosus Sjogren's syndrome Scleroderma Polymyositis/dermatomyositis Mixed connective tissue disease	Psoriasis Inflammatory bowel disease

Emergency Situations

Clinicians should be aware of several potential emergency situations that can occur in the setting of RA or the SPAs (**Table 7.7**). First and foremost, these patients are at increased risk for septic arthritis because (1) degenerative joints provide a safe haven for infectious bacteria, (2) synovitis causes increased vascularity such that hematogenous seeding of joints is more likely to occur in inflamed joints, (3) patients are likely to be on immunosuppressive therapy or have prosthetic joints, and (4) patients with PsA may have compromised skin integrity.[10] Suspicion for septic arthritis should be raised in a patient with RA or an SPA who presents with an inflamed monoarthritis but otherwise has well-controlled disease. Systemic symptoms may not be present, especially in patients on immunosuppressive medications, including low-dose steroids. In this setting, blood cultures and joint fluid analysis (including gram stain and culture) are warranted.

Table 7.7   Rheumatologic Emergencies in Rheumatoid Arthritis and the Spondyloarthropathies

CONDITION	FEATURES
Septic arthritis (RA or SPA)	Swollen inflamed joint out of proportion to other articular disease activity, especially in immunosuppressed patients.
Cervical spine disease (RA or SPA)	Cervical myelopathy manifesting as paresthesias and hyper-reflexia, often in the setting of long-standing disease. In RA, this occurs secondary to synovitis at the atlantoaxial interface. In SPA, myelopathy may indicate fracture of cervical spine to create a pseudoarthrosis. Potential neurosurgical emergency. May require fiber-optic intubation.
Cricoarytenoiditis (RA)	Presents as hoarseness and can cause laryngeal spasm and acute airway obstruction. Potential surgical emergency. May require fiber-optic intubation.
Cauda equina syndrome (SPA)	Central canal impingement of the cauda equina presenting as rapidly progressive lower extremity weakness, saddle anesthesia, hyporeflexia, and bladder/bowel retention.
Cardiac tamponade (RA)	Hemodynamic instability secondary to large chronic exudative pericardial effusion. May require pericardiocentesis.
Vasculitis (RA)	Many potential presentations, but mononeuritis multiplex or glomerulonephritis represent conditions that require emergent intervention.
Vasculitis, aortitis (SPA)	Aortic insufficiency or rupture secondary to chronic transmural inflammation. Potential cardiothoracic surgical emergency.
Scleromalacia (RA)	Ocular pain secondary to inflammation and thinning of sclera. May perforate orbit. Ophthalmologic emergency.
Macrophage activation syndrome or hemophagocytic syndrome (juvenile rheumatoid arthritis)	Causes marked systemic inflammation with hepatosplenomegaly and pancytopenia. Ferritin levels markedly elevated. Diagnosed by biopsy of affected tissue (e.g., bone marrow, liver, etc.).

Other rheumatic emergencies may arise in patients with RA or SPAs. Cervical spine disease may lead to atlantoaxial subluxation in patients with RA or fracture (with pseudo-arthrosis on plain film) in patients with SPAs. Patients may present with myelopathic findings or simply neck pain. Passive flexion–extension plain films of the neck are the most cost-effective modality to identify these complications of cervical spine disease. Further, spine instability may not be recognized when the patient is lying recumbently for magnetic resonance imaging (MRI) or computer tomography (CT) scan. In patients with RA or an SPA, cervical spine disease should be considered prior to any procedure that requires intubation. Patients with RA are also at risk for cricoarytenoiditis, which can also complicate intubation. In patients with cervical spine instability, spinal fusion may be necessary.

Additional emergency situations may arise in patients with RA and SPAs. Often, these patients have disease that has been long-standing or difficult to control. The SPAs have been associated with vasculitis of the proximal aorta. In RA, large pericardial effusions can lead to cardiac tamponade if unrecognized. Chronic scleritis may cause scleromalacia with threatened perforation of orbit. Small vessel vasculitis may present simply as leukocytoclastic vasculitis of the skin, but involvement of peripheral nerves (mononeuritis multiplex) or kidney (glomerulonephritis) may require more emergent intervention with immunosuppressive or cytotoxic agents. Macrophage activation syndrome (MAS), also known as the hemophagocytic syndrome, is a rare, highly inflammatory state that is usually limited to patients with systemic onset juvenile rheumatoid arthritis (JRA), but has been described in adults.[11] Patients present with fever, pancytopenia, fibrinolysis, and hepatosplenomegaly, which can lead to multiorgan failure. Ferritin may be markedly elevated, and diagnosis is made by biopsy of bone marrow, liver, or other affected organ. Despite aggressive immunosuppressive therapy, mortality rates are high.

DIAGNOSTIC STUDIES

Laboratory Tests

In RA and the SPAs, laboratory tests may be used to facilitate diagnosis or to guide treatment (**Table 7.8**). These tests should be performed in the appropriate clinical setting to maximize specificity, because no single laboratory test is yet diagnostic for RA or the SPAs. Approximately 80% of patients with RA will have elevated levels of RF or anti-CCP antibodies in the serum, but that leaves a substantial portion of patients who remain seronegative. The presence of these autoantibodies generally predicts a more aggressive disease course, but titers do not necessarily fluctuate with treatment response. Elevated antinuclear antibodies (ANAs) are common in patients with RA, but their presence is a nonspecific finding, because elevated ANAs exist in many other autoimmune connective tissue disorders as well (Table 7.1). RF, anti-CCP, and ANA tests are discussed in greater detail in Chapter 2.

The SPAs are generally described as seronegative diseases that do not have a known autoantibody signature. Class I major histocompatibility complex (MHC) genes that encode for human leukocyte antigen (HLA) B27 proteins have been associated with spinal arthritis in patients with SPA. HLA-B27 testing is controversial, however, and often not helpful. High background rates of HLA-B27 positivity in the general population reduce the specificity of a positive test, and most individuals with HLA-B27 do not develop spondylitis.

Table 7.8   Laboratory Tests in the Diagnosis and Management of Inflammatory Arthritis

CONDITION	LABORATORY TEST
Rheumatoid arthritis	Rheumatoid factor Anti-CCP antibodies Antinuclear antibody
Spondyloarthropathies	HLA-B27 in selected situations
Systemic inflammation (potentially useful in disease management)	Anemia of chronic disease Leukocytosis Thrombocytosis Elevated erythrocyte sedimentation rate (ESR) Elevated C-reactive protein (CRP) Elevated ferritin Elevated haptoglobin Elevated complements

Patients with active RA or an SPA often demonstrate laboratory abnormalities related to inflammation (Table 7.8). These changes are nonspecific, but provide some diagnostic utility when trying to distinguish inflammatory from mechanical joint disease in the appropriate clinical setting. The complete blood count (CBC) may reveal anemia of chronic disease, leukocytosis, and thrombocytosis. The erythrocyte sedimentation rate (ESR) is often elevated (although rarely >100 mm/hr). There is also typically an elevation in other acute phase reactants: C-reactive protein (CRP), ferritin, haptoglobin, and complements. Although diagnostically nonspecific, acute phase reactants serve a more important role in guiding drug management, because these values often fluctuate in relation to disease activity. In clinical trials, the ESR or CRP is included in most of the various outcome measurements that are used to determine drug efficacy.[12] Acute phase reactants are often elevated in the various SPAs as well, but it is not unusual for patients with SPA to show no elevation of acute phase reactants despite aggressive disease.

Imaging Studies

Musculoskeletal imaging studies are useful in both the diagnosis and management of patients with RA or SPAs. Each modality has its advantages and disadvantages (**Table 7.9**). Plain film radiography continues to be the mainstay of imaging because of rapid interpretation, low cost, and high prognostic value. In patients with RA and peripheral manifestations of an SPA, abnormalities in plain films follow a rather characteristic series of changes, although the tempo of change may vary from one patient to another (**Table 7.10**). Soft tissue swelling and periarticular osteopenia are the earliest radiologic signs of inflammatory arthritis. These early changes may be followed by joint space narrowing and marginal erosions, which indicate cartilage loss and bone resorption, respectively. Radiologic joint subluxation and ankylosis are late findings indicative of destructive disease. Mirroring clinical findings, radiologic changes in patients with RA tend to occur at the metacarpophalangeal (MCP) and proximal interphalangeal (PIP) joints of the hand and the metatarsophalangeal (MTP) and PIP joints of the feet, whereas the SPAs primarily affect the PIP and distal interphalangeal (DIP) joints of the hands and feet. One goal of therapy is to retard progression of radiologic damage in patients with inflammatory arthritis. Of note, patients with seropositive RA are at greater risk for developing erosive and destructive changes than seronegative RA patients.[13]

Table 7.9   Musculoskeletal Imaging Techniques: Advantages and Disadvantages

Technique	Advantages	Disadvantages
Plain films	Low cost Readily available	Poor soft tissue resolution Some radiation exposure
MRI	Excellent soft tissue resolution Detects preradiographic synovitis	High cost Limited availability Gadolinium contrast infusion
CT scan	Excellent bone resolution Can be used to direct procedures	Intermediate cost Moderate radiation exposure Moderate soft tissue resolution
Bone scan	Total body imaging May reveal subclinical disease	Intermediate cost Findings are often nonspecific
Ultrasound	Good soft tissue resolution Identifies synovitis and erosions Can be used to direct procedures	Intermediate cost Operator dependent

Table 7.10   Radiologic Changes in Peripheral Inflammatory Arthritis, Spondylitis, and Sacroiliitis

Peripheral Arthritis	Spondylitis	Sacroiliitis
Soft tissue swelling	Squaring of vertebral bodies	Joint sclerosis
Periarticular osteopenia	Syndesmophytes	Joint erosions
Joint space narrowing	Ligament calcification	Joint space narrowing
Marginal erosions	Fracture (pseudoarthrosis)	Joint space widening
Secondary osteoarthritis	Ankylosis	Ankylosis
Ankylosis		

In the SPAs, a different spectrum of radiographic changes is observed in the spine and sacroiliac (SI) joints when compared to peripheral joints (Table 7.10). In the spine, squaring of the vertebral bodies is an early change. Later changes include bridging syndesmophytes, calcification of the anterior longitudinal ligament, and ankylosis with resultant "bamboo spine." A pseudoarthrosis represents an unstable fracture through a vertebral body and may be a surgical emergency (detailed above). Pelvic radiographs may reveal changes at the sacroiliac (SI) joints that are highly specific for SPAs. Plain films may show erosions or sclerosis early, whereas joint space narrowing, widening, and ankylosis are later changes (Table 7.3). An anterior–posterior plain film of the pelvis also allows visualization of the hip joints, which are not infrequently involved in the SPAs. Providing 30 degrees of cephalad angulation on hip imaging allows for isolation of the SI joints (Ferguson view) and also reduces exposure of the gonads to radiation.

More advanced imaging studies are gaining a greater foothold in the diagnosis and management of patients with RA and the SPAs.[14] MRI reveals the greatest anatomic detail for most musculoskeletal structures, but it may not be readily available and carries a high expense. In addition to providing detail about the structural integrity of tendons and ligaments, MRI may reveal preradiographic evidence of inflammation: bone marrow edema, synovial thickening, tenosynovitis, joint effusion, cartilage defects, or early bone erosions. CT scan is ideal for defining boney abnormalities and can be used to guide interventional procedures. It carries risks of radiation exposure and intravenous (IV) contrast dye. Radionucleotide bone scans may reveal uptake at sites of inflammation, although changes may be nonspecific or difficult to interpret. Musculoskeletal ultrasound (US) is an emerging technique that permits visualization of the joint and surrounding soft tissue structures. It is highly operator-dependent, but it allows for dynamic examination of pathology without any radiation exposure or IV contrast risk. US can detect preradiographic erosions, and the power Doppler feature may detect the hypervascularity of synovitis. US may also be used to direct procedures.

Arthrocentesis

In the diagnostic workup of inflammatory arthritis, arthrocentesis is often unnecessary because the clinical setting, laboratory workup, and radiographic findings are more than sufficient to establish a diagnosis. Arthrocentesis is used primarily to rule out other causes of joint complaints, including noninflammatory processes, microcrystalline disease (e.g., gout or pseudogout), and septic arthritis. Synovial fluid should be tested for white blood count (WBC), differential WBC, crystals (polarized light microscopy), and microorganisms (gram stain and culture).

In RA and the SPAs, actively swollen joints usually demonstrate inflammatory synovial fluid (WBC >1500 cells/mm^3) consisting primarily, but not exclusively, of neutrophils (50–90%). When synovial fluid WBC is >50,000 cells/mm^3 or has >90% neutrophils, microcrystalline disease and septic arthritis are more likely disease entities.

In a patient with known RA or an SPA, noninflammatory joint fluid (WBC <1000 cells/ mm^3) should prompt consideration of partially-treated disease, internal derangement of a joint (e.g. ligament or meniscus injury), secondary degenerative OA in an affected joint, or a sympathetic effusion related to juxta-articular pathology (e.g., avascular necrosis). Arthrocentesis also provides a modality for directly targeting corticosteroid therapy in patients with autoimmune inflammatory arthritis (discussed below).

ESTABLISHING A DIAGNOSIS

As mentioned before, a diagnosis of RA or an SPA is made based on a combination of clinical presentation, laboratory findings, and radiographic imaging. Inflammatory arthritis should be strongly suspected when a patient presents with acute or subacute onset arthralgias, morning stiffness, functional deficit, and objectively warm, swollen joints on exam. In this setting, acute phase reactants (e.g., ESR or CRP) may be elevated, which would corroborate exam findings. Arthrocentesis may be performed to confirm the presence of inflammatory joint fluid or to rule out microcrystalline disease or septic arthritis. Serologic analysis for RF, anti-CCP antibodies, and ANAs are often useful to clarify a diagnosis, but they are not diagnostic in and of themselves. Plain film radiographic imaging is unlikely to demonstrate erosive or destructive changes in the early stages of inflammatory arthritis, but may show juxta-articular osteopenia or periarticular swelling. In unclear settings, MRI and ultrasound are more sensitive for synovitis. Any of these clinical scenarios should also prompt an expedited referral to a rheumatologist for diagnostic workup and initiation of immunomodulatory therapy.

TREATMENT

For many years, analgesics and corticosteroids were the only treatment options available for patients with inflammatory arthritis. Although these medications continue to serve important functions, the past two decades have seen great strides in our understanding of the pathophysiology of inflammatory arthritis. These advances have made possible the introduction of many newer therapeutic agents that are known collectively as DMARDs. This section outlines therapeutic strategies and treatment objectives for patients with inflammatory arthritides. Much of the discussion focuses on treatment of RA, for which there is a greater body of knowledge than that of the SPAs, which are also addressed. Chapter 16 provides much greater detail about the specific antirheumatic drugs, their mechanisms of action, dosing regimens, and toxicity profiles.

Reducing joint pain, swelling, and stiffness is an important short-term goal of antirheumatic therapy. Although this objective may be met through use of nonsteroidal anti-inflammatory drugs (NSAIDs), corticosteroids, and narcotic analgesics, these agents have well-established toxicities when used chronically (Chapter 16). In patients with RA, systemic corticosteroids are often rapidly effective in doses of only 5 to 10 mg daily prednisone (or equivalent). Intra-articular injection of corticosteroids is an alternative means to deliver therapy directly to a single involved joint, but this approach is impractical for most polyarticular disease. For unclear reasons, the SPAs are traditionally more refractory to systemic or intra-articular corticosteroids.

Corticosteroids and NSAIDs do not sufficiently address the overarching long-term treatment goal: disease remission as measured by retarding radiographic joint damage, restoring functionality, and maximizing quality of life. It is well established that early introduction of DMARDs under the supervision of a rheumatologist best allows for these long-term goals to be achieved.[3] In addition, DMARDs should also reduce the need for chronic corticosteroid therapy and its cumulative toxicities. For these reasons, corticosteroids are more likely to be used as a bridge therapy to treat a patient's immediate symptoms while introducing DMARDs, which often have a later onset of action.

In the treatment of inflammatory arthritis, there is no "one size fits all" approach, and many factors influence therapeutic decision making. The treating rheumatologist must balance established benefits of an adequate treatment regimen against potential toxicities of the various agents in order to maximize efficacy while limiting risk. Chapter 16 details relative and absolute contraindications for the various DMARDs, such as avoiding methotrexate in patients with severe renal insufficiency, liver diseases, or pregnancy. Although the more potent DMARDs tend to have the more serious potential side effects, most DMARDs are generally well tolerated when closely managed by rheumatologists and primary care providers with appropriate laboratory monitoring.

Minimizing medication toxicity is of paramount importance, but so is matching the immunomodulatory potency of a DMARD regimen to the severity of disease in order to avoid chronic undertreatment (or overtreatment) of the inflammatory process. Disease remission is the treatment goal, but patients should not be unduly exposed to excessive medication toxicity. In this regard, it is helpful to prognosticate aggressiveness of disease based on clinical presentation, imaging, and laboratory tests.

Small-Molecule DMARDs

Hydroxychloroquine (HCQ) and sulfasalazine (SSZ) are generally considered the mildest and best-tolerated of the DMARDs. On their own, either of these agents may adequately control disease activity in patients with an indolent presentation, normal radiographs, preserved function, normal or mildly elevated inflammatory markers, or seronegative serology (RF or anti-CCP negative). In contrast, the more potent DMARDs are warranted for patients who present with more severe symptoms, steroid refractoriness, early radiographic joint damage, marked functional disability, high inflammatory markers, or seropositive RF or anti-CCP serology. These patients often require rapid dose escalation of antimetabolite DMARDs (methotrexate and leflunomide), early introduction of biologic DMARDs, and combination DMARD therapy. Any and all of these approaches may be necessary to induce disease improvement, which can often be done safely and effectively with close monitoring. More potent agents are also indicated for patients who fail less effective therapies. Gold and azathioprine are two other DMARDs that are used infrequently in patients with inflammatory arthritis (see Chapter 16). Their usage is often limited to patients who are unable to tolerate other DMARDs or are unresponsive to other therapies.

For patients with moderately to severely active RA, methotrexate (MTX) is widely accepted as the benchmark DMARD to which all others are compared. It is a potent antimetabolite drug that is typically used in doses of 15 to 25 mg once weekly in oral or injectable formulations. Once-weekly dosing is crucial to avoid serious bone marrow aplasia, which is associated with more frequent dosing. Side effects of MTX can often be reduced by supplementation with either folic acid or leucovorin. Leflunomide is another drug with similar efficacy and toxicity profile as MTX. It is an oral medication dosed at 10 to 20 mg once daily. Additional information for both of these agents, including detailed side effects, can be found in Chapter 16. Routine blood counts and liver function testing are used to monitor for bone marrow and hepatic toxicities of these drugs, which are absolutely contraindicated in patients who are pregnant or attempting to conceive. MTX and leflunomide both require dose adjustment for impaired renal function and should be used with great caution or avoided entirely in patients with marked renal impairment.

Biologic DMARDs

The late 1990s saw the advent of biologic agents for the treatment of RA and SPAs. These new DMARDs have revolutionized treatment goals, and disease remission is attainable in a substantial proportion of patients. Choosing to add a biologic drug should be dictated by the aggressiveness of a patient's inflammatory arthritis, risk for toxicity, and availability of the drugs. These agents and their various side effects are discussed in greater detail in Chapter 16.

In patients who tolerate small-molecule DMARDs but continue to demonstrate moderate-to-severe active inflammatory arthritis, additional therapy is indicated, usually the addition of biologic DMARDs. These drugs often can be added safely to existing small-molecule therapy for an additive antirheumatic effect without undue toxicity. In other situations, biologic agents may need to be substituted for small-molecule DMARDs when patients do not tolerate the latter. Currently, biologic drugs should not be used together in combination, because there appears to be little additive benefit and a clearly increased risk of serious infection.[15] It should be noted that, for unclear reasons, small-molecule DMARDs are rarely beneficial in patients with spinal manifestations of the SPAs, whereas biologic DMARDs very effectively relieve symptoms.

The most widely used, extensively studied, and best understood class of biologic DMARDs inhibits the proinflammatory cytokine tumor necrosis factor alpha (TNFα).

Five anti-TNF drugs are currently available in the United States: infliximab, etanercept, adalimumab, golimumab, and certolizumab. Like all biologic DMARDs, anti-TNF drugs are administered via parenteral means, although dosing regimens vary (Chapter 16). These medications improve symptoms of inflammatory arthritis, reduce serologic markers of inflammation (e.g., CRP), improve quality of life, and restore functional status. Interestingly, inhibition of radiographic progression of joint disease is seen in patients with RA and peripheral SPAs, but not in those with spinal manifestations of the SPAs.

TNF antagonists are generally well tolerated, but multiple studies have shown that the risk of serious bacterial infection or atypical opportunistic infection is increased in patients taking these drugs. Bacterial pneumonia, soft tissue infection, joint infection, or urinary tract infections may be potentially life-threatening if not recognized or addressed early. Further, providers should have a low threshold for further diagnostic testing for opportunistic pathogens in patients who are not responding to traditional empiric antibacterial therapy. Patients taking these agents have an increased risk for mycobacterial infections (tuberculous and nontuberculous), fungal infections, and other atypical infections. Preventative measures are effective; patients should be immunized against pneumococcus and tested for latent tuberculosis prior to starting anti-TNF antagonist therapy. Latent tuberculosis should be treated appropriately. Patients should also receive a yearly immunization against influenza.

Other biologic agents have other mechanisms of action. Abatacept is a fusion protein of cytotoxic T-lymphocyte antigen 4 (CTLA4) and a modified Fc portion of human immunoglobulin Cγ1. It blocks T cell activation by binding to and blocking the costimulatory molecules CD80 and CD86 on antigen presenting cells. Abatacept is effective in the treatment of RA, although the time-to-onset of action may not occur for 3 to 4 months in some patients. Rituximab is a chimeric human–mouse anti-CD20 monoclonal antibody that depletes CD20-expressing B cells. It was originally developed as B cell ablative therapy for the treatment of B cell lymphomas. Its uses have been extended to RA, where it is used in patients who have failed TNF-inhibitor therapy. The consequences of chronic B cell depletion are mostly unknown. Anakinra is a synthetically produced IL1 receptor antagonist (IL1-Ra) that antagonizes receptor binding of IL1, another proinflammatory cytokine. As a therapeutic agent for the treatment of RA, it is only mildly effective and is therefore rarely used. Tocilizumab is a monoclonal antibody that binds to and blocks the receptor for IL6, another proinflammatory cytokine. It has recently been approved in the United States for use in RA, and has shown benefit in Phase III clinical trials.

Collectively, the biologic DMARDs have been an incredibly important advance in the treatment of RA and the SPAs, and many patients have benefitted greatly from their usage. All biologic DMARDs are much more expensive than small-molecule agents, however, and this has added a cost-benefit analysis to decision making about treatment. Still unresolved is the issue of whether one biologic agent is better than another in the treatment of chronic inflammatory arthritis. Studies comparing different biologic agents in head-to-head clinical trials are lacking.

Additional Measures

Nonpharmacologic modalities play an important role in the management of RA and the SPAs. Physical therapy and occupational therapy are important adjunctive measures that improve patient function, reduce disability, and maintain musculoskeletal conditioning independent of drug activities. For patients with deforming changes of inflammatory arthritis, mechanical devices may assist with a range of activities, including ambulatory mobility, gross motor skills, and fine motor function.

Surgery remains an important interventional option in patients with inflammatory arthritis. For patients with a persistent monoarthritis, synovectomy (arthroscopic or open approach) often provides very effective short-term relief. Long-term benefits are variable because synovitis returns in a substantial proportion of patients. In some patients with destructive joint changes from chronic inflammatory arthritis, no amount of DMARD therapy can eliminate pain or restore meaningful function. In these instances, prosthetic joint replacement may be warranted. Replacements of hips or knees are often the most successful modality to improve ambulation and reduce pain. Replacements of elbows or shoulders are more difficult to perform technically, but results are very good with the newer implants and improved surgical expertise. Surgical fusion of the ankle or wrist can reduce pain without too much loss of function. Sometimes surgical realignment of MCPs or MTPs is warranted. Spinal fusion in patients with spondylitis or cervical RA is often reserved for those with spine-threatening fracture or cervical instability. Overall, surgical correction of deficits should be considered on a case-by-case basis. Patients should not wait until overly impaired from a functional standpoint prior to surgical evaluation, especially because better preoperative functional status correlates with improved postoperative rehabilitation.

CROSS-SPECIALTY ISSUES: CARDIOVASCULAR DISEASE AND CANCER

Many recent lines of evidence point to a likely contribution of chronic inflammation in the pathophysiology of atherosclerotic cardiovascular disease[16] and possibly cancer.[17] Macrophages and other inflammatory infiltrates are present in unstable lipid-rich atherosclerotic plaques. Patients with a chronically elevated CRP may be at increased risk for cardiovascular mortality. Patients with RA demonstrate increased risks for cardiovascular disease and cancer in many epidemiologic studies, some of which antedate modern biologic therapy. These associations in the SPAs may also exist but are less well-studied.

An increase in certain cancers, including non-Hodgkin's lymphoma and possibly lung cancer, has been seen in RA patients. These cancer risks appear to be increased in patients with RA independent of treatment, and it remains unclear whether TNF inhibitors affect this risk in a beneficial or detrimental direction.[18] It is important that primary care physicians consider cardiovascular risk when evaluating patients with RA. In this regard, age-appropriate screening for cardiovascular disease and cancer should be emphasized in all patients with RA and not relegated to the "back burner" of care.

SUMMARY

The inflammatory arthritides represent a diverse spectrum of chronic disease entities that collectively cause significant morbidity and disability, especially when considering that patients tend to be afflicted during their most productive work years. No single symptom, examination feature, laboratory test, or diagnostic study can be used to diagnose these conditions. Rather, a combination of these features must be considered. A prompt diagnosis and referral to a rheumatologist allows for early therapeutic intervention. Oral small-molecule DMARDs, such as methotrexate, represent first-line treatment options for inflammatory arthritis. Biologic DMARDs provide excellent alternatives when patients cannot tolerate or are not responding to small-molecule agents. The biologic DMARDs can be used either as monotherapy or in combination with small-molecule DMARDs. Combination therapy of a biologic DMARD plus methotrexate is generally better than methotrexate or a biologic DMARD alone. When monitored carefully, DMARDs can be safely used to reduce symptoms, retard radiographic joint destruction, restore function, and improve quality of life. Long term, these reductions in morbidity translate into increased productivity, reduced need for total joint replacement, and possibly lower mortality.

◇◇◇◇◇◇◇◇◇◇◇◇

REFERENCES

1. Arnett FC, Edworthy SM, Bloch DA, et al. The American Rheumatism Association 1987 revised criteria for the classification of rheumatoid arthritis. *Arthritis Rheum.* 1988;31:315–324.

2. Goie The HS, Steven MM, van der Linden SM, Cats A. Evaluation of diagnostic criteria for ankylosing spondylitis: a comparison of the Rome, New York and modified New York criteria in patients with a positive clinical history screening test for ankylosing spondylitis. *Br J Rheumatol.* 1985;24:242–249.

3. Emery P, Breedveld FC, Dougados M, Kalden JR, Schiff MH, Smolen JS. Early referral recommendation for newly diagnosed rheumatoid arthritis: evidence based development of a clinical guide. *Ann Rheum Dis.* 2002;61:290–297.

4. Helmick CG, Felson DT, Lawrence RC, et al. Estimates of the prevalence of arthritis and other rheumatic conditions in the United States. Part I. *Arthritis Rheum.* 2008;58:15–25.

5. Feitsma AL, van der Helm-van Mil AH, Huizinga TW, de Vries RR, Toes RE. Protection against rheumatoid arthritis by HLA: nature and nurture. *Ann Rheum Dis.* 2008;67(Suppl 3):61–63.

6. Costenbader KH, Feskanich D, Mandl LA, Karlson EW. Smoking intensity, duration, and cessation, and the risk of rheumatoid arthritis in women. *Am J Med.* 2006;119:501–509.

7. Callahan LF. The burden of rheumatoid arthritis: facts and figures. *J Rheumatol.* 1998;53:8–12.

8. Khan MA. Update on spondyloarthropathies. *Ann Intern Med.* 2002;136:896–907.

9. Kaarela K, Tiitinen S, Luukkainen R. Long-term prognosis of monoarthritis. A follow-up study. *Scand J Rheumatol.* 1983;12:374–376.

10. Ostensson A, Geborek P. Septic arthritis as a nonsurgical complication in rheumatoid arthritis: relation to disease severity and therapy. *Br J Rheumatol.* 1991;30:35–38.

11. Singh S, Samant R, Joshi VR. Adult onset Still's disease: a study of 14 cases. *Clin Rheumatol.* 2008;27:35–39.

12. Felson DT, Anderson JJ, Boers M, et al. American College of Rheumatology. Preliminary definition of improvement in rheumatoid arthritis. *Arthritis Rheum.* 1995;38:727–735.

13. Edelman J, Russell AS. A comparison of patients with seropositive and seronegative rheumatoid arthritis. *Rheumatol Int.* 1983;3:47–48.

14. Ostergaard M, Pedersen SJ, Dohn UM. Imaging in rheumatoid arthritis—status and recent advances for magnetic resonance imaging, ultrasonography, computed tomography and conventional radiography. *Best Pract Res Clin Rheumatol.* 2008;22:1019–1044.

15. Weinblatt M, Combe B, Covucci A, Aranda R, Becker JC, Keystone E. Safety of the selective costimulation modulator abatacept in rheumatoid arthritis patients receiving background biologic and nonbiologic disease-modifying antirheumatic drugs: A one-year randomized, placebo-controlled study. *Arthritis Rheum.* 2006;54:2807–2816.

16. Ridker PM, Solomon DH. Should patients with rheumatoid arthritis receive statin therapy? Arthritis Rheum. 2009;60:1205–1209.

17. Llorca J, Lopez-Diaz MJ, Gonzalez-Juanatey C, Ollier WE, Martin J, Gonzalez-Gay MA. Persistent chronic inflammation contributes to the development of cancer in patients with rheumatoid arthritis from a defined population of northwestern Spain. *Semin Arthritis Rheum.* 2007;37:31–38.

18. Kaiser R. Incidence of lymphoma in patients with rheumatoid arthritis: a systematic review of the literature. *Clin Lymphoma Myeloma.* 2008;8:87-93.

CHAPTER 8

Polymyalgia Rheumatica and Giant Cell Arteritis

Susan Y. Ritter, MD, PhD

OVERVIEW

Polymyalgia rheumatica (PMR) is a clinical syndrome affecting older individuals that causes aching and stiffness in the shoulder, neck, and pelvic girdle regions and is associated with elevated inflammatory markers. It responds well to low doses of prednisone and may be a limited condition or a herald of another condition. One of the other conditions associated with PMR is giant cell arteritis.

Giant cell arteritis (GCA) is a vasculitis that affects medium- and large-sized arteries in older individuals. Another commonly used term for this condition is *temporal arteritis*. The classically affected locations of this vasculitis include the temporal arteries of the skull and branches of the aorta, although other arterial involvement has rarely been described. In distinction from PMR, treatment of GCA requires higher doses of steroids for longer periods of time.

There appears to be a relationship between these two conditions. Evidence for an association is that PMR symptoms are common in patients with GCA, and a subset of patients with PMR symptoms will go on to develop GCA. Further insight into the exact relationship is not entirely clear at this point, although they may share a similar pathophysiology.

EPIDEMIOLOGY

Both PMR and GCA typically affect individuals after the age of 50. In fact, the incidence continues to increase with age such that approximately 90% of the cases occur in individuals older than age 60. There is a slightly increased incidence in women compared to men. Studies assessing incidence of GCA in different countries show the highest rates in Scandinavian countries, with an incidence of 20 per 100,000, and the lowest rates in Asian countries, with an incidence of 1.47 per 100,000 in Japan. Even within Europe, there is a higher incidence in northern latitudes compared to southern latitudes. PMR is at least twice as common as GCA and has a similar age range and ethnicity.

PATHOLOGY/PATHOGENESIS

Little is known about the pathology associated with PMR. A synovitis can be seen in involved joints, but generally pathologic specimens are not used to confirm the diagnosis of PMR. In contrast, the diagnosis of GCA is often made by temporal artery biopsy. The classical pathologic description of GCA is a granulomatous inflammatory infiltrate of lymphocytes, macrophages, and multinucleated giant cells at the intima-media junction, which is associated with disruption of the internal elastic lamina. However, the histologic changes seen in a biopsy sample can be varied with granulomatous lesions, nonspecific white cell infiltration, or intimal fibrosis. These changes are often segmental in nature, and thus biopsy of a large segment of the temporal artery is advisable so as to not miss skip lesions.

Studies to assess the mechanism behind GCA suggest that dendritic cells within the adventitia-medial border of the artery are involved in disease initiation. It is not clear what the exact trigger is for disease initiation. However, it does seem that dendritic cells become activated via toll-like receptors and produce chemokines that recruit T cells and macrophages into the vessel wall. The CD4+ T cells then produce cytokines, such as interferon gamma, interleukin-1 (IL-1), and interleukin-6 (IL-6), that perpetuate the inflammatory cascade and lead to further damage to the vessel wall. Over time, matrix metalloproteinase and other locally produced factors cause damage to the vessel and promote remodeling and fibrosis. These pathologic changes and inflammatory mediators have been seen in PMR as well as in GCA. However, it appears that interferon gamma is not produced in the PMR tissues, perhaps leading to a milder vascular phenotype. Many of the systemic manifestations of both GCA and PMR are likely related to the inflammatory cytokines produced in the lesions.

COMMON CLINICAL MANIFESTATIONS

The clinical manifestations of PMR and GCA overlap. The most classic symptom in PMR is aching or stiffness in the shoulder, neck, and pelvic girdles. PMR symptoms can be present in just the shoulders or just the pelvic region in some patients and can start unilateral then become bilateral in others. The pain is worse with movement, at night, and is often described in the muscles around the joints and not necessarily the joints themselves. There may be morning stiffness with gelling after inactivity, similar to rheumatoid arthritis. Symptoms such as bursitis, carpal tunnel, peripheral arthritis, and swelling of the hands and wrists have all been described. PMR symptoms have been described in as many as 50% of GCA patients. However, GCA symptoms differ in that fever is more common, as is new-onset headache, affecting two-thirds of patients. The headache can be in the region of the temporal arteries or anywhere in the head, and patients may describe scalp tenderness with brushing or combing the hair. Visual loss is the most feared complication of GCA. The visual loss can be caused by narrowing of the posterior ciliary arteries or retinal artery occlusion. A fundoscopic examination may be able to detect early changes in blood flow to the optic disc. Amaurosis fugax is reported in 15% in some series and can precede permanent visual loss. Once visual loss has occurred, it is unlikely for sight to return in that eye. Finally, if GCA affects more than just the cranial vessels, there may be asymmetric pulses, and thus a vascular assessment and bilateral blood pressure measurement is important in disease diagnosis.

Table 8.1   Common Symptoms of Polymyalgia Rheumatica Versus Giant Cell Arteritis

POLYMYALGIA RHEUMATICA	GIANT CELL ARTERITIS
Aching and stiffness in the neck, shoulders, and pelvic girdle	Fever
Weight loss	New-onset headache
Low-grade fever	Jaw claudication
Depression	Aching/stiffness of PMR
Fatigue	Temporal tenderness
Anorexia	Diplopia, amaurosis fugax, or visual loss

DIAGNOSIS

Laboratory Findings

Both PMR and GCA are characterized by elevated inflammatory markers. Typically, the erythrocyte sedimentation rate (ESR) is at least 40 mm/h in PMR and can be even higher (>50 mm/h) in GCA. However, PMR can occur with a normal ESR. Some studies suggest this can be seen up to 20% of patients. C-reactive protein (CRP) is also frequently elevated in both PMR and GCA. In some cases, the CRP may be elevated but the ESR is normal. In this case, following the CRP during disease monitoring can be helpful to assess response to therapy. Other, less specific findings include an anemia of chronic disease and occasional mild elevations in liver enzymes.

Imaging

At present, imaging studies are not sufficient for diagnosis of either PMR or GCA, but it is possible that with improvements in technology they may eventually play a role in diagnosis. In PMR, ultrasound, magnetic resonance imaging (MRI), and fluorodeoxyglucose positron emission tomography (PET) have demonstrated synovitis and bursitis of the shoulder or hip girdles in almost all patients. In GCA, ultrasound may be able to show a hypoechoic halo around the lumen of an inflamed temporal artery. High-resolution MRI can show enhancement of the temporal arteries or aortic arch. A fluorodeoxyglucose PET can show the extent of extracranial vasculitis. Conventional angiography can show stenosis of the great vessels and may be helpful if GCA is strongly suspected but the temporal artery biopsy is negative.

Tissue Examination

Tissue biopsy is not useful for the diagnosis of PMR. However, tissue diagnosis remains the gold standard for diagnosis of giant cell arteritis. The classical pathologic features associated with GCA have been described above. Temporal artery biopsy is a simple outpatient procedure that is associated with very little clinical morbidity. Biopsies are typically performed by general surgeons, vascular surgeons, or neuro-ophthamologists. The biopsy is done around the hairline, such that visible scarring is rare. However, aspects of temporal artery biopsy deserve special attention. Due to potential risk of visual loss or stroke in patients with active vasculitis, treatment should be initiated as soon as the diagnosis of giant cell arteritis is suspected. Treatment prior to biopsy is unlikely to affect the result of the biopsy so long as the biopsy is performed within 1 to 2 weeks of commencing glucocorticoid therapy. Due to the skip lesions typically seen in biopsy specimens, a longer arterial biopsy is preferred. It is our preference that a specimen of at least 2 cm be obtained so as to capture the highest yield. Sometimes inflammation is seen in one artery but not another. For this reason, bilateral biopsies are sometimes performed. However, the additional yield obtained from biopsy of the contra lateral side is on the order of 3 to 12%, depending on the series. Typically, if one side is more tender or grossly abnormal by exam, it is reasonable to biopsy one side. If the diagnosis is less clear and one would like with the maximum degree of certainty to rule in or out a diagnosis, then a bilateral biopsy can be performed.

Differential Diagnoses

PMR has several mimics. One of the most important to assess is rheumatoid arthritis. For this reason, it is reasonable to assess for rheumatoid factor and anti-cyclic citrullinated peptide antibodies in patients with PMR symptoms and peripheral arthritis. Spondyloarthritis is another possible cause of axial symptoms and elevated ESR, but assessment for enthesitis, dactylitis, or uveitis can help differentiate this from PMR and these entities usually occur in a younger age group. Calcium pyrophosphate dihydrate deposition disease (CPPD) disease is common in elderly females and may cause pain and limited range of motion of affected joints. Rarely, polyarticular gout can cause similar symptoms as well. Typically, synovial fluid analysis and radiographic studies can help in the assessment of this entity. Finally, fibromyalgia is commonly in the differential diagnosis for periarticular joint pain. However, it is the author's opinion that fibromyalgia rarely presents after the age of 50, and patients with fibromyalgia generally do not have morning joint stiffness and elevated inflammatory markers. Myositis typically causes proximal muscle weakness rather than pain and is associated with elevated muscle enzymes. Other vasculitides can be considered, such as ANCA-associated vasculitis and Takayasu's arteritis, but they can often be differentiated by location of involved vessels, antibodies, or age. Finally, PMR symptoms have been described as a paraneoplastic phenomenon in some malignancies, such as renal cell carcinoma.

Table 8.2 Classification Criteria for Giant Cell Arteritis

AGE ≥50 YEARS AT DISEASE ONSET
New headache
Temporal artery tenderness or decreased pulsation unrelated to peripheral vascular disease
ESR ≥50 mm/h
Temporal artery biopsy showing vasculitis with mononuclear cell infiltration or granulomatous inflammation

Note: A patient is said to have GCA if at least three of the five criteria are present. Sensitivity is 93.5%, and specificity is 91.2%.

Table 8.3 Comparison of Three Diagnostic Criteria for PMR[1-3]

RESEARCHERS	CRITERIA
Chuang and colleagues	Age ≥50 years; bilateral aching and stiffness for 1 month of two regions: neck, shoulders/arms, hips/thighs; ESR ≥40 mm/h; exclusion of other diagnoses
Healey	Persistent pain involving two of the following: neck, shoulders, pelvic girdle; morning stiffness lasting >1 hour; rapid response to prednisone (≤20 mg/day); absence of other diseases; age >50 years; ESR >40 mm/h
Bird	Bilateral shoulder pain/stiffness; onset of illness within 2 weeks; initial ESR >0 mm/h; morning stiffness >1 hour; age >65 years; depression and/or weight loss; bilateral upper arm tenderness (need three or more criteria)

TREATMENT AND CLINICAL COURSE

Prednisone is the mainstay of PMR therapy. An initial dose of 10 to 20 mg per day is often sufficient to resolve the musculoskeletal pain within days. The response to prednisone is so dramatic that it frequently can be used as a diagnostic test (see Healey criteria in Table 8.3). Some patients will have breakthrough symptoms and require twice daily dosing. After symptoms have resolved, the daily dose of prednisone can be tapered every 2 to 4 weeks. Generally, the taper from 10 to 20 mg per day to 5 mg per day is well tolerated. Unfortunately, tapering below 5 mg per day can be more challenging, and thus the taper may need to be slowed to 1 mg per month after this point. Most patients require prednisone therapy for 1 to 2 years. Patients should be assessed for recurrent PMR symptoms, development of GCA symptoms, and ESR and/or CRP levels during the taper. ESR and CRP levels may be variable over time, and thus elevation of inflammatory markers in the absence of symptoms is not considered a relapse or reason to increase the steroid dose. A slow prednisone taper is advised, as faster tapering can lead to a higher rate of relapse. Few options are available for patients who are intolerant of prednisone. Methotrexate has been tried with some success as a steroid-limiting agent, but trials of other anti-inflammatory drugs have not been successful. In addition, there are some case reports of hydroxychlorquine used in PMR as a steroid-sparing agent. Thought should be given to minimizing the risks of steroid therapy, such as diabetes and osteoporosis, and appropriate monitoring and prophylaxis considered for osteoporosis.

In GCA, higher dose corticosteroids are necessary to reverse the vasculitis. Typically, a dose of prednisone 1 mg/kg per day is initiated, although lower doses (40 to 60 mg) may be sufficient in some patients. Higher dose intravenous methylprednisolone (1000 mg for 3 days) is commonly used in patients with recent or impending visual loss. This initial dose of prednisone is generally given for up to 4 weeks until inflammatory markers have normalized and symptoms have resolved. At this point, the steroids can be tapered gradually. By approximately 3 months after diagnosis, a dose of 10 to 15 mg per day (PMR range) can often be achieved. Some patients are able to discontinue steroid therapy in 1 to 2 years, but other may continue to need low doses for longer periods of time. Monitoring during therapy includes assessment of extracranial vessels, monitoring for aortic insufficiency, and consideration of vascular imaging, such as chest imaging and monitoring for thoracic and abdominal aortic aneurysms. Calcium, vitamin D, and bisphosphonates should be considered in patients with osteopenia or osteoporosis. Steroid-sparing agents have been tried in GCA with varying success. The most promising is methotrexate; low doses have been shown to minimize the total dose and duration of prednisone and decrease relapse. However, some studies have not shown a benefit to adding methotrexate to steroids for GCA. Methotrexate can be considered as an adjunctive agent to steroids in a patient who is intolerant of high-dose glucocorticoids or who develops severe steroid-related side effects. Therapies such as azathioprine, cyclosporine, and infliximab have not been successful in this disease. Finally, patients with GCA are at increased risk of cardiovascular and cerebrovascular thrombotic events. Several studies have shown a decreased risk for ischemic complications in patients on aspirin therapy, and thus all patients with GCA consider low-dose aspirin therapy.

◇◇◇◇◇◇◇◇◇◇◇◇

REFERENCES

1. Chuang T-Y, et al. Polymyalgia rheumatica: a 10-year epidemiologic and clinical study. *Ann Intern Med.* 1982;97:672–80.
2. Healey LA. Long-term follow-up of polymyalgia rheumatica: evidence for synovitis. *Semin Arthritis Rheum.* 1984;13:322–28.
3. Bird HA, et al. An evaluation of criteria for polymyalgia rheumatica. *Ann Rheum Dis.* 1979;38:434–39.

◇◇◇◇◇◇◇◇◇◇◇◇◇◇◇◇◇◇◇◇◇◇

SUGGESTED READINGS

Boyev LR, Miller NR, Green WR. Efficacy of unilateral versus bilateral temporal artery biopsies for the diagnosis of giant cell arteritis. *Am J Ophthalmol.* 1999;128(2):211–215.

Breur GS, Nesher G, Nesher R. Rate of discordant findings in bilateral temporal biopsy to diagnose giant cell arteritis. *J Rheumatol.* 2009;36(4):794–796.

Lee MS, Smith SD, Galor A, Hoffman GS. Antiplatelet and anticoagulant therapy in patients with giant cell arteritis. *Arthritis Rheum.* 2006;54(10):3306–3309.

Levine SM, DB Hellmann. Giant cell arteritis. *Curr Opin Rheumatol.* 2002;14:3–10.

Mahr AD, Jover JA, Spiera RF, et al. Adjunctive methotrexate for treatment of giant cell arteritis: an individual patient data meta-analysis. *Arthritis Rheum.* 2007;56(8):2789–2794.

Ma-Krupa W, Jeon MS, Spoerl S, Tedder TF, Goronzy JJ, Weyand CM. Activation of arterial wall dendritic cells and breakdown of self-tolerance in giant cell arteritis. *JEM.* 2004;199(2):173–183.

Mukhtyar C, Guillevin L, Cid MC, et al. EULAR recommendations for the management of large vessel vasculitis. *Ann Rheum Dis.* 2009;68:318–323.

Nesher G, Berkun Y, Mates M, Baras M, Rubinow A, Sonnenblick M. Low-dose aspirin and prevention of cranial ischemic complications in giant cell arteritis. *Arthritis Rheum.* 2004;50(4):1332–1337.

Salvarani C, Cantini F, Hunder GG. Polymyalgia rheumatic aand giant-cell arteritis. *Lancet.* 2008;372:234–245.

Weyand CM, Goronzy JJ. Giant-cell arteritis and polymyalgia rheumatica. *Ann Intern Med.* 2003;139:505–515.

Yilmaz A, Arditi M. Giant cell arteritis: takes two t's to tango. *Circ Res.* 2009;104:425–427.

CHAPTER 9

Systemic Lupus Erythematosus

Martin A. Kriegel, MD, PhD
Bonnie Bermas, MD

OVERVIEW

Systemic lupus erythematosus (SLE) is a complex, polygenic, multisystem disease with varying manifestations between and within patients. It is considered the prototype of a systemic autoimmune disease. Lupus erythematosus can be classified as systemic lupus erythematosus (SLE; 70%), skin-limited (cutaneous lupus; 15%), drug-induced (5%), and as an overlap syndrome, such as mixed connective tissue disease (MCTD) or undifferentiated connective tissue disease (10%). In this chapter, we will discuss the pathogenesis, clinical and laboratory features, and general treatment principals of SLE with emphasis on practical issues relevant to the general physician.

EPIDEMIOLOGY, GENETICS, AND PATHOGENESIS

The prevalence of systemic lupus erythematosus varies from 40 to over 400 cases per 100,000 persons depending on ethnicity, being less common among Northern Europeans and more prevalent among African Americans. The highest rates have been found in Afro-Caribbeans and Sioux Native Americans. Sex also plays a major role; 90% of patients with SLE are female. SLE is as common as 1 in 250 African American females. In Caucasians, lupus is seen in 1 of 1000 females, but only in 1 of 10,000 males. The sex difference in lupus prevalence is diminished in cases emerging before puberty and in the elderly. However, SLE most commonly evolves during the reproductive years, when females are significantly overrepresented.

Mortality from SLE has improved considerably over the last 50 years due to treatment advances. In the past, the 4-year survival had been as low as 50%, but currently the 15-year survival rate is at least 80%. It has long been recognized that mortality in SLE is distributed in a bimodal pattern, with earlier deaths caused by complications of the disease itself and infections versus later deaths occurring because of associated cardiovascular disease.

The pathogenesis of SLE is complex, and multiple factors, including genes, environment (e.g., smoking), hormones, and immune dysregulation contribute to disease expression and severity. Subclinical autoimmunity (i.e., serologic evidence of autoreactivity without clinical manifestations) has been shown to precede overt disease for years, even decades. Specific autoantibodies progressively accumulate before the onset of SLE. Multiple genetic studies, as well as more recent large-scale genomic scans, have elucidated major genetic susceptibility loci, gene polymorphisms, and potential candidate genes in SLE. **Table 9.1** lists disease-promoting genes that have been implicated in the pathogenesis of SLE.

Table 9.1   Potential or Confirmed Candidate Genes from Genetic or Genome-Wide Association Studies of SLE patients*

GENE(S)	PROPOSED ROLE IN PATHOGENESIS
STAT4, IRF5	Cytokine signaling, "interferon signature"
FCGR2A/B	Immune complex clearance, lymphocyte activation
CTLA-4, PDCD1	T cell costimulation and tolerance
HLA-DRB1	Antigen presentation, adaptive immunity
C1q, C2, C4 (deficiencies)	Dysregulated apoptosis, immune complex clearance
PTPN22	Altered lymphocyte signaling and activation
BANK1	B cell signaling and hyperreactivity
ITGAM	Neutrophil/monocyte adherence, phagocytosis

* STAT4, signal transducer and activator of transcription 4; IRF5, interferon regulatory factor 5; FCGR2A/B, Fc-gamma receptor IIA/B; CTLA-4, cytotoxic T-lymphocyte antigen-4; PDCD1, programmed cell death 1; HLA-DRB1, human leukocyte antigen DRB1; PTPN22, protein tyrosine phosphatase N22; BANK1, B cell scaffold protein with ankyrin repeats 1; ITGAM, integrin alpha M.

Environmental exposures such as ultraviolet light, infections (especially viral), and certain drugs (including hydralazine, procainamide, methyldopa, and tumor necrosis factor blockers) induce or exacerbate SLE through various mechanisms. One theory of how these triggers cause SLE is that increased apoptosis or defective clearance of apoptotic blebs, such as those resulting from viral infection, leads secondarily to release of nuclear autoantigens (including DNA, RNA, and associated binding proteins). For instance, complement is involved in clearing apoptotic debris, and rare monogenic complement deficiencies cause SLE in the majority of these cases. Extracellular abundance of nuclear antigens triggers highly conserved innate immune receptors. Enhanced signaling via these toll-like receptors (TLR) 3, 7, and 9, which recognize DNA and RNA compounds, contributes to secretion of interferon-alpha from specialized dendritic cells, the so-called plasmacytoid dendritic cells. This important antiviral cytokine seems to be crucial in linking innate and adaptive immunity/autoimmunity. Genetic associations with aberrant signaling molecules of the interferon pathway have been found (Table 9.1). A so called "interferon signature" was recently identified in some SLE patients. IFN-alpha is also induced during viral infections, which might explain exacerbations during intercurrent illnesses. Strategies to block IFN-alpha are currently in development.

Once these nuclear antigens are presented to autoreactive T and B cells, systemic autoimmunity can develop after an adaptive immune response has been generated. Deficiency of suppressor T cells and T cell resistance to tolerization are both signs of impaired peripheral T cell tolerance, likely contributing to the pathogenesis of SLE. Uninhibited, self-reactive CD4+ T cells can activate B cells to produce autoantibodies against a diverse array of antigens, supporting the theory that polyclonal B cell activation is a hallmark of SLE. Autoantigens released during cell death include double-stranded (ds) DNA, which is the prototypic antigen targeted in SLE. However, dsDNA antibodies are present only in 70 to 80% of patients, so this cannot be the only explanation. Antinuclear antibodies (ANA) are present in up to 100% of persons with SLE. However, ANA can be seen in a variety of other diseases and are not specific to SLE. Among the various autoantibodies, anti-dsDNA antibodies have been shown to be pathogenic by fixing complement and subsequently leading to glomerular damage. Low complement levels of C3 and C4 are indicators of active lupus nephritis (see below). In summary, various aberrations in the innate and adaptive immune system contribute to the pathogenesis of SLE in a genetically susceptible person exposed to the appropriate external or endogenous triggers.

CLINICAL SPECTRUM

SLE can affect nearly every organ of the body. Many important signs, symptoms, and laboratory abnormalities have been summarized in the American College of Rheumatology (ACR) criteria (**Table 9.2**). The proposed ACR classification is based on 11 criteria. For clinical studies, a person is said to have SLE if 4 or more of the 11 criteria are present, serially or simultaneously, during any interval of observation.

Table 9.2   Revised 1982 ACR Criteria for SLE[1,2]

CRITERION	DEFINITION
Malar rash	Fixed erythema, flat or raised, over the malar eminences, tending to spare the nasolabial folds
Discoid rash	Erythematous raised patches with adherent keratotic scaling and follicular plugging; atrophic scarring may occur in older lesions
Photosensitivity	Skin rash as a result of unusual reaction to sunlight, by patient history or physician observation
Oral ulcers	Oral or nasopharyngeal ulceration, usually painless, observed by physician
Arthritis	Nonerosive arthritis involving two or more peripheral joints, characterized by tenderness, swelling, or effusion
Serositis	a) Pleuritis—convincing history of pleuritic pain or rubbing heard by a physician or evidence of pleural effusion *OR* (b) Pericarditis—documented by ECG or rub or evidence of pericardial effusion

(continues)

Table 9.2   Revised 1982 ACR Criteria for SLE,[1,2] cont'd

CRITERION	DEFINITION
Renal disorder	(a) Persistent proteinuria greater than 0.5 grams per day or greater than 3+ if quantitation not performed *OR* (b) Cellular casts—may be red cell, hemoglobin, granular, tubular, or mixed
Neurologic disorder	(a) Seizures—in the absence of offending drugs or known metabolic derangements; e.g., uremia, ketoacidosis, or electrolyte imbalance *OR* (b) Psychosis—in the absence of offending drugs or known metabolic derangements; e.g., uremia, ketoacidosis, or electrolyte imbalance
Hematologic disorder	(a) Hemolytic anemia—with reticulocytosis *OR* (b) Leukopenia—less than 4000/mm^3 total on two or more occasions *OR* (c) Lymphopenia—less than 1500/mm^3 on two or more occasions *OR* (d) Thrombocytopenia—less than 100,000/mm^3 in the absence of offending drugs

Immunologic disorder	(a) Anti-DNA—antibody to native DNA in abnormal titer
	OR
	(b) Anti-Sm—presence of antibody to Sm nuclear antigen
	OR
	(c) Positive finding of antiphospholipid antibodies based on
	  (1) an abnormal serum level of IgG or IgM anticardiolipin antibodies
	  (2) a positive test result for lupus anticoagulant using a standard method
	    OR
	  (3) a false-positive serologic test for syphilis known to be positive for at least 6 months and confirmed by *Treponema pallidum* immobilization or fluorescent treponemal antibody absorption test

Antinuclear antibody	An abnormal titer of antinuclear antibody by immunofluorescence or an equivalent assay at any point in time and in the absence of drugs known to be associated with "drug-induced lupus" syndrome

Adapted from Tan EM, et al., Arthritis Rheum. 1982;25:1271, and Hochberg MC, Arthritis Rheum. 1997;40:1725.

The criteria presented in Table 9.2 can assist in making a diagnosis of SLE, but they should be used with caution because they were developed for use in clinical studies. In cases of severe organ system involvement, a person can present with fewer than 4 of the 11 ACR criteria yet clinically be considered to have SLE. The diagnosis of SLE thus depends on a combination of signs and symptoms that might be unique in individual SLE patients.

POSITIVE ANTINUCLEAR ANTIBODIES

It is important to note that a positive antinuclear antibodies (ANA) test does not make the diagnosis of SLE. Although it is necessary (at least 98% of persons with SLE have this antibody), it is not sufficient, because fewer than 10% of individuals with a positive ANA fulfill the criteria for SLE. Interpretation of a positive ANA can be misleading, for instance, in patients with thyroid disease, because they frequently have a nonspecific positive titer. Common scenarios of ANA positivity in the absence of systemic rheumatic diseases are provided in **Tables 9.3** and **9.4**.

Table 9.3 Organ-Specific Autoimmune Diseases Associated with a Positive ANA Test

DISEASE	SENSITIVITIES FOR ANA
Autoimmune hepatitis	60–90%
Thyroid disease (Grave's disease/Hashimoto's thyroiditis)	50%
Idiopathic pulmonary hypertension	40%
Primary biliary cirrhosis	10–40%

Table 9.4 Nonautoimmune Conditions Associated with a Positive ANA test

DISEASE/CONDITION	EXAMPLES
Viral infection	HIV, hepatitis B or C, Epstein-Barr virus
Bacterial infection	Subacute bacterial endocarditis
Mycobacterial infection	Tuberculosis
Hematologic malignancy	Acute myelogenous leukemia
Age	20–40% over age 65
Healthy individuals	Up to 10% of the general population
Drugs	Anti-tumor necrosis factor agents

CLINICAL SIGNS AND SYMPTOMS

Constitutional Symptoms

Constitutional symptoms are among the most common manifestations of lupus in persons with SLE. Malaise and fatigue are present in up to 90%, fever in over 50%, and weight loss in roughly 25%. However, these symptoms are very nonspecific and require exclusion of infectious or hemato-oncologic causes.

Mucocutaneous and Vascular System

A classic manifestation of SLE is the malar rash in a "butterfly" pattern sparing the nasolabial folds (see **Figure 9.1**). The characteristic distribution is thought to be related to those areas that receive the most exposure to UV light. UV sensitivity is a hallmark of lupus. In general, the presence of a malar rash strongly suggests SLE but is found only in roughly one-third of patients and can often be confused with other skin diseases, such as rosacea (although rosacea usually involves the nasolabial folds). If a skin biopsy is performed, the so-called "lupus band test" is characteristically positive on pathology in about 60% of those tested. A band of localized immunoglobulins at the dermal–epidermal junction is seen on direct immunofluorescence.

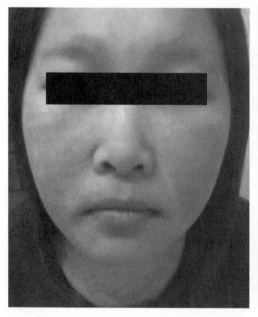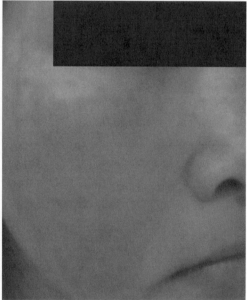

Figure 9.1

Malar rash in a 23-year-old Asian female with SLE. This patient is suffering from an acute flare with marked proteinuria and acute cutaneous lesions also on her upper chest and back. A corticosteroid cream has just been applied to the face.

Oral ulcers are less common than the malar rash. Oral ulcers frequently are located on the buccal mucosa or hard palate and are typically painless. Dry mouth as part of the so-called sicca symptoms is typically a complaint with secondary Sjogren's syndrome. Patchy alopecia can also occur in lupus. Various other skin findings, including urticarial or bullous lesions, have been described. Papulosquamous, annular, plaque-like, or scarring lesions in sun-exposed areas are part of the spectrum of cutaneous lupus and must be differentiated from SLE. Chronic cutaneous lupus only rarely evolves into the systemic form, but subacute cutaneous lupus develops systemic features in about 5 to 15% of patients over 10 years.

Vascular phenomena in SLE include Raynaud's syndrome and livedo reticularis. These are frequently associated with antiphospholipid syndrome. Severe Raynaud's phenomenon can lead to fingertip ulcers. Finally, cutaneous vasculitis involving the small and medium vessels can occur in SLE.

Musculoskeletal System

Diffuse joint pain and myalgias are very common and difficult to differentiate from secondary fibromyalgia. Nonerosive arthritis is seen in about half of all SLE patients. Rarely (less than 5 to 10% of patients), chronic inflammation of the tendons can lead to so-called Jaccoud's arthritis, causing subluxations and ulnar deviation of the finger joints. These deformities are due to ligamentous laxity and typically are not associated with erosions, as seen in rheumatoid arthritis. Chronic steroid treatment increases the risk for osteoporosis and avascular necrosis (AVN). Acute onset of hip or shoulder pain in a patient with longstanding systemic lupus erythematosus should always alert the clinician to consider AVN, given that it is more common in this patient population even in the absence of corticosteroid use.

Kidney and Urogenital System

The kidney is affected in 30 to 40% of SLE patients. Lupus nephritis (LN) can be a life-threatening manifestation of SLE and requires intensive immunosuppressive therapy in at least half of all cases. Hematuria, proteinuria, and casts are typically found on urinalysis with sediment. A renal biopsy is frequently necessary to classify the disease and assess indices of activity versus chronicity. LN is categorized based on the histology. Treatment regimens can vary substantially depending on which class the patient's kidney disease falls into. The International Society of Nephrology and Renal Pathology Society (ISN/RPS) defines six classes of LN (**Table 9.5**). This classification is based on morphologic lesions, extent and severity of involvement, mesangial or subepithelial deposition of immune complexes, and activity versus chronicity.

Table 9.5   Classification of Lupus Nephritis Based on the International Society of Nephrology and Renal Pathology

CLASS	PATHOLOGY/DESCRIPTION
I	Minimal mesangial (mesangial deposits by immunofluorescence)
II	Mesangial proliferative (mesangial deposits by light microscopy; mesangial hypercellularity)
III	Focal proliferative (less than 50% glomerular involvement) III (A): active (focal proliferative) III (A/C): active/chronic (focal proliferative and sclerosing) III (C): chronic inactive (focal sclerosing)
IV	Diffuse proliferative (over 50% glomerular involvement) IV-S (A) or IV-G (A): active (diffuse segmental or global proliferative) IV-S (A/C) or IV-G (A/C): active/chronic (diffuse segmental or global proliferative) IV-S (C) or IV-G (C): chronic inactive (diffuse segmental or global sclerosing)
V	Membranous (subepithelial deposits)
VI	Advanced sclerosis (over 90% sclerotic glomeruli)

Nephrotic syndrome as seen in class V LN is associated with an increased risk for thrombosis; this can be substantially higher if the patient is also positive for antiphospholipid antibodies. Renal vein thrombosis is another manifestation in SLE patients and is associated with secondary antiphospholipid syndrome. Patients with class III/VI LN carry at least a 5 to 10% risk of requiring hemodialysis after 10 years of disease duration. Low C3 and elevated anti-dsDNA antibodies correlate with disease activity in these categories and are helpful in distinguishing a flare from other causes of acute renal failure. Standard measures taken in patients with chronic kidney disease in general should also apply to patients with LN. For instance, weight, blood pressure, electrolytes, and urinary protein should be monitored regularly in patients with LN. The protein-to-creatinine ratio is helpful in assessing the severity of class V nephritis over time, although the less convenient 24-hour urinary protein collection would be more accurate.

Hematopoietic System

Lymphadenopathy and mild-to-moderate splenomegaly are signs of immune activation and can occasionally be appreciated on physical examination. Scattered small mediastinal or abdominal lymph nodes are frequently found on computed tomography (CT) imaging studies of patients with active disease. Moderate-size lymphadenopathy should prompt further investigations, because lymphomas should not be missed, especially in patients previously treated with cytotoxic agents. Histiocytic necrotizing lymphadenitis, or Kikuchi's disease, is also on the differential diagnosis of a patient with large cervical lymph nodes and systemic symptoms but without sufficient criteria for SLE.

Cytopenias due to autoimmune phenomena are part of the ACR criteria provided in Table 9.2. Autoimmune hemolytic anemia is prevalent in up to 10% of SLE patients. Signs of hemolysis and a positive Coombs' test are typically present. Other causes of anemia, most notably anemia of chronic disease, frequently coexist. Leukopenia and lymphopenia are very common features in SLE. Idiopathic thrombocytopenic purpura (ITP) associated with SLE requires treatment if profound or if clinically relevant thrombocytopenia develops. Thrombotic thrombocytopenic purpura (TTP) is rare, but can be missed if renal and CNS involvement is mistaken for manifestations from primary disease. A blood smear to assess for schistocytes is essential to rule out this life-threatening entity. Prompt initiation of plasmapheresis is indicated if TTP is confirmed.

Cardiopulmonary System

Serositis is very common in SLE, and small pleural or pericardial effusions are incidentally found in over 50% of patients. Associated pleuritic chest pain can be bothersome for patients. Large pleural effusions requiring drainage are rare but have been reported. If thoracentesis is performed, exudative pleural fluid is typically obtained. However, these findings are largely nonspecific except if so-called "LE cells" are found on Wright stain. LE cells are polymorphonuclear leukocytes containing large phagocytosed nuclei. In general, ANA and complement levels should not be checked in a pleural fluid sample, because they reflect serum levels.

Interstitial lung disease can be seen in SLE and also in MCTD or secondary Sjogren's syndrome. A CT scan of the chest may reveal ground-glass opacities or a honeycomb pattern; the latter finding suggests irreversibility. Pulmonary hypertension is defined by a mean pulmonary artery pressure above 50 mm Hg on right heart catheterization; it is often missed in the early stages until dyspnea is progressive. MCTD, scleroderma overlap, or antiphospholipid syndrome should be considered in patients with pulmonary hypertension. The 6-minute walk test, an electrocardiogram (ECG), and pulmonary function tests are part of the initial workup. A right heart catheterization is necessary to confirm the diagnosis and help with treatment decisions based on reversibility after vasodilator challenge.

Acute lupus pneumonitis is a rare manifestation (less than 5 to 10%) that can present acutely with fever. It must be differentiated from pneumonia. It is associated with high mortality, but responds to high-dose steroids if administered promptly. Pulmonary hemorrhage occurs even less frequently (under 1%), but carries a poor prognosis if hemoptysis is fulminant. Pulmonary emboli are frequently seen in patients with secondary antiphospholipid syndrome, which requires lifelong anticoagulation.

The cardiovascular system is also involved in SLE. The most common manifestation is pericarditis. Lupus myocarditis is seen in fewer than 5 to 10% of patients. Rarely, a cardiomyopathy can develop after years of hydroxychloroquine use. Sterile, so-called Libman-Sacks, endocarditis can lead to peripheral embolization, including to the CNS, with subsequent neurologic sequelae. The majority of patients with Libman-Sacks endocarditis have antiphospholipid antibodies.

One of the leading causes of mortality in patients with systemic lupus erythematosus is the increased risk of coronary artery disease (CAD). This increased relative risk is significant in younger patients. Although medications and classic atherosclerotic risk factors are important mediators of this phenomenon, the disease itself, with concomitant inflammation, plays a role as well. Based on several recent trials, elevated C-reactive protein (CRP) levels even in patients without underlying SLE or other rheumatic disease appear to be a marker for greater risk for cardiovascular disease.

Nervous System and Eye

Any part of the central and peripheral nervous system can be involved in SLE patients. Up to 30% of patients develop some lupus-related neurologic symptoms. Signs and symptoms vary widely, from minor cognitive dysfunction to seizures, extensive strokes, or quadriplegia from transverse myelitis. Defined neuropsychiatric syndromes in SLE are summarized in **Table 9.6**.

Table 9.6   Neuropsychiatric Syndromes in SLE

NEUROLOGIC CENTRAL MANIFESTATIONS	PSYCHIATRIC CENTRAL MANIFESTATIONS	PERIPHERAL MANIFESTATIONS
Aseptic meningitis	Acute confusional state	Guillain-Barre syndrome
Cerebrovascular disease	Anxiety disorder	Autonomic neuropathy
Demyelinating syndrome	Cognitive dysfunction	Mononeuropathy
Headache	Mood disorder	Myasthenia gravis
Movement disorder	Psychosis	Cranial neuropathy
Myelopathy		Plexopathy
Seizure disorder		Polyneuropathy

General inflammation, cytokines, and specific targeting of neural tissues by antibodies or immune cells are thought to be intrinsic mechanisms in neuropsychiatric lupus. However, infections, medications, and cerebrovascular disease from accelerated atherosclerosis are common secondary causes of neuropsychiatric signs and symptoms. Secondary antiphospholipid antibody syndrome is another condition that can lead to various neurologic sequelae in SLE patients, primarily via thromboembolic disease. Posterior reversible encephalitis syndrome (PRES) has been associated with poorly controlled hypertension or certain immunosuppressive drugs in SLE (most notably cyclosporine). It has been speculated that effective hypovolemia from protein loss in LN as well as inflammation-induced endothelial cell dysfunction might be more directly involved in the pathogenesis of PRES, which is an increasingly recognized entity in SLE.

The differentiation of lupus cerebritis from infectious meningitis can be difficult. Brain imaging might not be conclusive, and a lumbar puncture is almost always necessary. Oligoclonal bands and increased synthesis of IgG is typically seen in the cerebrospinal fluid (CSF) analysis. The presence of LE cells in the CSF is highly specific for CNS lupus. Antineuronal or antiribosomal P antibodies are frequently found in the CSF of patients with CNS lupus. However, ribosomal P antibodies are also found in high frequency in SLE patients with septic meningitis. General findings on CSF analysis in CNS lupus are listed in **Table 9.7**.

Table 9.7   Neuropsychiatric Syndromes in SLE

CSF FINDING	PERCENT AFFECTED
Mild pleocytosis	20–35%
Elevated protein	25–50%
Normal glucose	>90%
Antineuronal antibodies	40–90%
Oligoclonal bands/high IgG index	20–80%
LE cells	Rare

CNS vasculitis is rare but can be seen early in the course of systemic lupus and needs to be treated aggressively. Cerebrovascular events are serious complications from lupus-associated ITP or TTP, as discussed in the section on the hematopoietic system. CNS bleeding secondary to thromboemboli warrants investigation of antiphospholipid antibody status and cryoglobulins.

Spinal cord involvement can occur from myelitis, vasculitis, or antiphospholipid syndrome. The latter two conditions can also affect the peripheral nervous system. Signs or symptoms from peripheral nervous system involvement can be seen in 10% of SLE patients. Examples of lupus-associated conditions specific to peripheral nervous system are Guillain-Barre syndrome, chronic demyelinating inflammatory neuropathy, and mononeuritis multiplex.

Various parts of the eye can also be involved in SLE patients. Secondary Sjogren's syndrome can cause severe keratoconjunctivitis sicca due to inflammation of the lacrimal glands. Mild dryness of the eyes is common in SLE patients with positive anti-SSA or anti-SSB. However, uveitis, retinal vasculitis, and optic neuritis are rare in systemic lupus. Drug-related toxicities should also be considered if patients complain of vision changes or other eye-related symptoms. Specifically, corticosteroid-induced glaucoma or cataracts and hydroxychloroquine-associated retinal deposits are to be considered (see section on treatment).

Gastrointestinal Tract and Liver

Nonspecific transaminitis is frequently seen in patients with a severe lupus flare exhibiting systemic symptoms. Hepatic granulomas, autoimmune hepatitis, and various SLE-related medications can also cause liver enzyme abnormalities. Small amounts of ascites are often found incidentally on imaging studies in patients with active SLE, frequently associated with serositis in the pleural and pericardial spaces. Nephrotic syndrome from class V nephritis can also contribute to ascites. Patients suffering from MCTD or overlap syndromes with scleroderma or inflammatory myositis may complain of dysphagia, which warrants further investigation. In younger patients, protein-losing enteropathies can present with large-volume diarrhea, rarely even as the initial symptom of SLE. Otherwise, involvement of the large or small bowel is exceedingly rare if not associated with other autoimmune diseases, such as ulcerative colitis or celiac disease. However, the occurrence of mesenteric vasculitis should not be missed, because it can be life-threatening and requires aggressive immunosuppression. Pancreatitis is rarely associated with systemic lupus. Concomitant treatment for SLE with azathioprine or steroids has been implicated in lupus pancreatitis, but is controversial. Finally, thromboembolic events from secondary antiphospholipid syndrome can affect various parts of the gastrointestinal tract or liver (e.g., mesenteric vein thrombosis, Budd-Chiari syndrome).

LABORATORY TESTING

A multitude of serologic studies supplement the diagnosis and monitoring of SLE. Disease subsets are often defined based on various autoantibody patterns. However, basic laboratory evaluations, including inflammatory markers; blood counts; renal function tests; and urinalysis, including sediment, are often of greater importance and should always be checked first if a flare or new-onset lupus is suspected.

Transaminases, muscle enzymes, coagulation studies, and thyroid function tests often are part of the initial workup. ECG, chest radiographs, or more sensitive imaging studies are indicated based on the various presenting signs or symptoms. This section focuses on SLE-related serologic tests and the role of complement.

Autoantibodies

ANA are the hallmark of SLE. The diagnosis of SLE should be questioned if there is not a history of ANA positivity. A few cases of ANA-negative lupus were described in the 1970s and 1980s, most likely due to insufficient substrates for testing. Since the availability of Hep-2 cells to assay for ANA, this entity is likely not to be described anymore. The ANA test, however, is not specific for SLE, because approximately 5 to 10% of healthy individuals can have a positive ANA, and the prevalence is even higher in the older population. In general, the higher the ANA titer, the more likely it is that the patient may develop a systemic autoimmune disease in the future. A variety of systemic rheumatic diseases are characterized by a positive ANA. The frequency of a positive ANA test in these disorders is provided in **Table 9.8**. In addition, several nonrheumatic (i.e., autoimmune, infectious, malignant) illnesses are associated with a positive ANA, as discussed previously.

Table 9.8 Systemic Rheumatic Diseases Associated with a Positive ANA Test

DISEASE	PERCENT
Drug-induced lupus (ANA+ by definition)	100%
Mixed connective tissue disease (defined by RNP positivity)	100%
Systemic lupus erythematosus	Up to 100%
Scleroderma	80%
Pauciarticular juvenile rheumatoid arthritis	70%
Inflammatory myositis	60%
Sjogren's syndrome	50%
Rheumatoid arthritis	40%

The staining pattern of ANAs (i.e., diffuse versus speckled, peripheral versus centromeric) suggests the presence of certain subtypes. Several laboratories now automatically check for so-called extractable nuclear antigens (ENAs) if the ANA test is positive. Therefore, the pattern of ANA staining has become less crucial over time, but it is still helpful in patients without defined subtypes. The most significant ENA subtype in SLE is the anti-dsDNA, which is very specific and correlates with active LN (class III/IV), as mentioned earlier.

Anti-Smith is only positive in about 10% of patients, but it is also highly specific for disease diagnosis. Anti-SSA/-SSB antibodies (also known as anti-Ro/-La) produce a speckled staining pattern and are commonly found in secondary Sjogren's syndrome and neonatal lupus and are particularly associated with skin manifestations in SLE or cutaneous lupus. They can also stain the cytoplasm, because the antigens are thought to shuttle between the nucleus and cytoplasm. Anti-SSA antibodies are particularly implicated in congenital heart block. Anti-SSA/-SSB antibodies are routinely screened for in pregnant lupus patients in order to predict neonatal complications.

Antiribonucleoprotein (RNP) antibodies often indicate the presence of MCTD. Anti-RNP antibodies are associated with Raynaud's phenomenon and pulmonary hypertension. In addition to anti-SSA/-SSB antibodies, antiribosomal P antibodies stain the cytoplasm where the ribosome is located. They are implicated in neuropsychiatric lupus and can also be measured in the CSF in addition to serum, as discussed in the section on nervous system involvement. The important autoantibodies are listed in **Table 9.9**.

Table 9.9   Antigen-Specific Nuclear/Cytoplasmic Autoantibodies and Their Prevalence in SLE

ANTIGENIC TARGET	PREVALENCE	ASSOCIATIONS/COMMENTS
dsDNA	40–60%	Active renal disease, hemolytic anemia
SSA (Ro)	30–40%	Cutaneous lesions, neonatal lupus
SSB (La)	10–15%	Neonatal lupus
Smith	10–20%	Very specific, CNS disease
U1-RNP	25–40%	Raynaud's, pulmonary hypertension, MCTD
Histone	20–90%	Nonspecific, 90% in drug-induced lupus
Ribosomal P (cytoplasmic)	10–40%	Psychosis, depression, renal disease

Antibodies directed against cells or extracellular components are also implicated in certain manifestations. **Tables 9.10** and **9.11** summarize their association with cytopenias, neurologic symptoms, antiphospholipid syndrome, and coagulopathies.

Table 9.10   Cellular Targets of Autoantibodies in SLE and Their Clinical Relevance

CELL TYPE	CLINICAL CONSEQUENCES
Red blood cells	Autoimmune hemolytic anemia
Platelets	Immune-mediated thrombocytopenia
Lymphocytes	Lymphopenia (disturbed immune homeostasis)
Granulocytes	Neutropenia, infection
Neurons	Neuropsychiatric lupus

Table 9.11   Extracellular Targets of Autoantibodies in SLE and Their Clinical Relevance

TARGET	CLINICAL CONSEQUENCES
Cardiolipin	Antiphospholipid syndrome, thrombosis
Beta-2 glycoprotein	Antiphospholipid syndrome, thrombosis
Prothrombin	Antiphospholipid syndrome, thrombosis

(continues)

Table 9.11   Extracellular Targets of Autoantibodies in SLE and Their Clinical Relevance, cont'd

TARGET	CLINICAL CONSEQUENCES
vWF antigen	Acquired von Willebrand's syndrome
Factor XI	Bleeding, coagulopathy

Other autoantibodies detected in SLE that are usually specific for other systemic autoimmune diseases include rheumatoid factor (RF), anti-cyclic citrullinated peptide (CCP), and anti-neutrophil cytoplasmic antibodies (ANCA). RF (typically IgM anti-IgG antibody directed against the Fc portion) is positive in about 30% of SLE patients. Its clinical significance in SLE is unclear, although overlapping cases with erosive, rheumatoid arthritis have been described. Anti-CCP antibodies are also rarely (<5%) positive in SLE despite their high specificity for rheumatoid arthritis. Finally, ANCA titers can occasionally be measured in SLE without any clinical association with vasculitis.

Complement

In addition to the various autoantibodies, monitoring of complement levels is very useful in detecting disease activity, particularly with regard to renal disease and autoimmune hemolytic anemia. The combination of rising anti-dsDNA antibodies and falling complement is a strong indicator for an evolving renal flare. The components C3 and C4 are usually followed to monitor disease activity. Some clinicians also check the total complement pathway (CH50), which includes these components. Some patients have persistently low complement levels despite recovery from a flare, possibly reflecting continuous low-level disease activity. In very rare cases, a genetic deficiency explains an isolated, chronically low complement component. Low complement levels in a SLE patient with longstanding nephrotic syndrome can occasionally also be due to severe protein loss as opposed to active disease. If C3 or C4 are higher than normal, they reflect likely nonspecific inflammation or infection, because complement factors are also acute phase reactants.

In summary, basic laboratory tests, including complete blood counts, electrolytes, creatinine, urinalysis, sedimentation rate, and CRP, usually are initially checked when evaluating a symptomatic SLE patient, but various autoimmune serologies and complement levels provide more detailed information about the severity and types of organs and tissues possibly involved during a flare.

TREATMENT

Treatment of SLE largely depends on whether the disease involves the major organs. Mild SLE that does not affect the organs and that is characterized by skin rashes, cytopenias, serositis, and mild arthritis can be managed with nonsteroidal anti-inflammatory drugs (NSAIDs), low doses of corticosteroids (less than 10 mg/day equivalent of prednisone), and hydroxychloroquine. More severe or organ-threatening disease needs to be treated with immunosuppressive and/or cytotoxic agents.

Nonsteroidal Anti-Inflammatory Drugs

A variety of NSAIDs are available for patients with mild SLE. They are used similarly with regards to frequency and dosing as in other rheumatic diseases. They are usually taken as needed, but for persistent symptoms they may be taken on a continuous basis. Constitutional symptoms, joint complaints, and serositis are typical indications for NSAIDs. Naproxen, diclofenac, ibuprofen, meloxicam, or similar agents can be used to control such symptoms. Allergies to sulfa components are more frequent in SLE patients compared to the general population. NSAIDs with a sulfa moiety (e.g., celecoxib) or sun-sensitizing effects should generally be avoided in susceptible patients. A proton-pump inhibitor or H2 blocker should be added in patients with epigastric complaints or prior history of gastrointestinal bleeding. This is especially recommended in patients on concomitant corticosteroids.

Antimalarial Agents

Evidence suggests that hydroxychloroquine may protect against more severe sequelae of SLE and therefore should be recommended for all patients with SLE unless there is a contraindication. Hydroxychloroquine is preferred over chloroquine, because it is thought to be less toxic. Hydroxychloroquine is usually started at 200 or 400 mg a day, with dosing kept under 6.5 mg/kg to avoid ocular toxicity. At least annual retinal exams are recommended because of the rare complication of retinal deposits causing potentially irreversible damage. However, fewer than 10% of patients experience retinal toxicity within 10 years. More common side effects include epigastric pain or abdominal cramping, diarrhea, flu-like symptoms, and headaches. Case reports of cardiomyopathy and conduction abnormalities have been described after prolonged treatment.

Glucocorticosteroid Therapy

Various topical steroid creams, lotions, and ointments (with increased absorption) are available on the market for cutaneous manifestations of SLE. Higher potency steroid creams should not be used for longer than 2-week periods, especially on the face given their local side effects, including skin atrophy and teleangiectasias.

Oral or intravenous glucocorticoids are very effective for acute management of organ involvement in SLE. Moderate-to-high doses (e.g., 0.5 to 1 mg/kg prednisone orally daily) are often necessary with a slow taper over 2 to 4 weeks. Intravenous pulse steroids are occasionally necessary in organ-threatening disease. Long-term therapy with corticosteroids should be kept at a safe dose below 7.5 mg of prednisone equivalent, if possible.

However, doses around 10 to 15 mg are often necessary to keep disease activity quiet. Ideally, long-term treatment with glucocorticoids should be avoided given the well-known toxicities, including loss of bone mineral density, steroid-induced diabetes, worsening of hypertension or atherosclerosis, gastrointestinal bleeding (particularly in combination with NSAIDs), avascular necrosis, cataracts, glaucoma, and changes in mood or sleep. A baseline bone mineral density is recommended in all patients on long-term steroid therapy (greater than 5 mg of daily prednisone equivalent for greater than 12 weeks). Weight-bearing exercises, a calcium-rich diet, oral calcium 1200 mg daily and vitamin D 800 IU daily are essential to prevent bone loss. In addition, postmenopausal women, elderly men, and younger male patients at risk should be started on a bisphosphonate for osteoporosis prevention (e.g., oral alendronate 35 mg weekly). Patients should sit upright and take these medications at least half an hour before breakfast in the morning to prevent reflux esophagitis. If gastroesophageal reflux is a problem, intravenous bisphosphonate therapy should be tried. The risk for osteonecrosis of the jaw is generally very low in patients who do not undergo major dental work.

Immunosuppressants

A steroid-sparing agent can be introduced in a patient requiring prolonged glucocorticoid therapy for persistently active disease. In addition, inability to control organ-threatening disease despite intravenous or oral glucocorticoids requires rapid institution of immuno-suppressive or cytotoxic agents. Severe class III, IV, or V nephritis is classically treated with intravenous pulse cyclophosphamide or mycophenolate mofetil. A commonly used cyclophosphamide regimen consists of 750 mg/m^2 on a monthly basis for 6 months, followed by quarterly pulses for 2 years, although a newer protocol developed in Europe with 500 mg/m^2 every 2 weeks for 12 weeks has been used with success. Serious infectious complications, infertility, bladder toxicity, and long-term induction of malignancies are obvious drawbacks of this therapy, although these side effects are less common with the European protocol. Mycophenolate mofetil titrated to 1500 mg twice daily may be as effective in inducing remission and avoids the risk of infertility. Mycophenolate mofetil should not be given in patients with significant renal impairment because it is cleared renally.

Cyclosporine in dosing at 3 mg/kg daily divided doses is effective in class V (membranous) nephritis. Azathioprine is another alternative for active renal disease and is also effective in liver and various other organ involvement. The thiopurine S-methyltransferase (TPMT) level should be checked prior to initiation of azathioprine in order to avoid excessive bone marrow toxicity in patients with heterozygous deficiency of this enzyme, which is prevalent in 10% of the population. More serious homozygous deficiency is only present in about 1%. The initial dose is usually 50 mg/day with uptitration to 150 mg/day over 2 weeks if blood counts remain stable. Cyclosporine and azathioprine may both be used during pregnancy, whereas cyclophosphamide and mycophenolate mofetil are contraindicated.

Leflunomide at 20 mg/day or methotrexate at similar doses used for rheumatoid arthritis (e.g., 15 to 20 mg/week with daily folic acid) are effective immunosuppressive agents for nonrenal manifestations, specifically arthritis and extensive cutaneous involvement. They are not indicated in organ-threatening SLE.

In general, regular monitoring with blood draws is warranted with use of any immunosuppressive drug. Complete blood counts and liver and kidney function are usually checked after the first month on a new immunosuppressant, and then every two to three months once a stable dose has been achieved with no significant side effects.

Other potential agents for LN or organ-threatening SLE include rituximab, a B cell-depleting antibody to the CD20 antigen (marking mature peripheral B cells), as well as abatacept, a CTLA4-Ig fusion protein, which blocks costimulation of lymphocytes. Abatacept is currently being tested in clinical trials after successful use in murine lupus models and in patients with rheumatoid arthritis. Infliximab, a chimeric TNF inhibitor, is also currently being studied in LN (class V), despite the potential of exacerbating SLE given several reports of drug-induced SLE after exposure to anti-TNF drugs.

General Health Measures

High-potency sunscreens or sunblocks are recommended to prevent flares triggered by excessive UV exposure. Vaccinations should be kept up-to-date; influenza and pneumococcal vaccinations are generally recommended in this patient population. Live vaccines (including nasal influenza vaccine) should be avoided once a patient is on immunosuppressants or on prolonged, moderate-to-high doses of corticosteroids (generally if on or above 20 mg of prednisone equivalent for over 12 weeks). Patients who have Raynaud's symptoms should dress in layers. Calcium channel blockers and topical nitropaste can be helpful in treating Raynaud's symptoms.

Treatment Regimens Based on Severity

Treatment of SLE depends largely on the severity of the disease. Mild SLE is characterized by constitutional symptoms, arthralgias, photosensitivity, and pleurisy. Moderate SLE is characterized by significant arthritis, cytopenias, pericardial or pleural effusions, or organ-involving disease, including myocarditis, cerebritis, and moderate proliferative or membranous LN (class III–V). Severe manifestations include refractory disease or life-threatening presentations, especially severe class III/VI/V SLE. **Table 9.12** summarizes the general treatment principles for mild, moderate, and severe SLE.

Table 9.12 Treatment of SLE Based on Disease Severity

SEVERITY	PHARMACOLOGIC THERAPY
Mild	NSAIDs; hydroxychloroquine; low doses of corticosteroids, taper over days to weeks
Moderate	Moderate-to-high doses of corticosteroids (up to 1 mg/kg/day prednisolone equivalent); taper over weeks to months; with or without introduction of a steroid-sparing agent early on (e.g., mycophenolate, azathioprine, cyclosporine, etc.)
Severe, life-threatening	Intravenous pulse corticosteroids, with or without intravenous pulse cyclophosphamide for 6 months; mycophenolate or azathioprine for maintenance therapy

SUMMARY

In summary, SLE is a systemic disorder predominantly affecting young women with a disproportionate disease burden on persons of African American, Latino, or Asian ethnicity. Disease manifestation ranges from mild to life-threatening. Improved disease management with use of immunosuppressants has vastly improved mortality.

◇◇◇◇◇◇◇◇◇◇◇◇

REFERENCES

1. Tan EM, Cohen AS, Fries JF, et al. Classification of systemic lupus erythematosus. *Arthritis Rheum.* 1982;25:1271–1277.

2. Hochberg MC. Updating the American College of Rheumatology revised criteria for systemic lupus erythematosus [letter]. *Arthritis Rheum.* 1997;40:1725.

◇◇◇◇◇◇◇◇◇◇◇◇◇◇◇◇◇◇◇◇

SUGGESTED READINGS

Firestein GS, et al. *Kelley's textbook of rheumatology,* 8th ed. New York: Elsevier Saunders; 2009.

Ginzler EM, Dooley MA, Aranow C, et al. Mycophenolate mofetil or intravenous cyclophosphamide for lupus nephritis. *N Engl J Med.* 2005;353:2219–2228.

Hochberg MC, et al. *Rheumatology,* 4th ed. New York: Elsevier; 2009.

Lahita RG. *Systemic lupus erythematosus,* 4th ed. New York: Elsevier, Academic Press; 2004.

Rahman A, Isenberg DA. Systemic lupus erythematosus. *N Engl J Med.* 2008;358:929–939.

Tsokos GC, Gordon PC, Smolen JS (eds.). *Systemic lupus erythematosus: a companion to rheumatology.* New York: Elsevier; 2007.

Wallace DJ. *Lupus: the essential clinician's guide.* New York: Oxford University Press; 2008.

Wallace DJ, Hahn BH. *Dubois' lupus erythematosus,* 7th ed. Philadelphia: Lippencott Williams and Wilkins; 2006.

CHAPTER 10

Antiphospholipid Antibody Syndrome

Martin A. Kriegel, MD, PhD
Bonnie Bermas, MD

OVERVIEW

Antiphospholipid antibody syndrome (APS) is defined as the presence of an antibody directed against phospholipids—anticardiolipin antibody or anti-β2 glycoprotein-I antibody—and/or a lupus anticoagulant in conjunction with thromboembolic events (venous or arterial) or pregnancy-related complications. Laboratory tests need to be positive on two occasions at least 12 weeks apart. Also, the clinical and/or laboratory features should not be separated by more than 5 years. The syndrome can occur in the presence of SLE as well as other autoimmune diseases (secondary APS) or as its own entity (primary APS).

EPIDEMIOLOGY AND PATHOGENESIS

Although low titers of antiphospholipid antibodies occur relatively often in the general population (up to 10%), moderate-to-high titers or a positive lupus anticoagulant test are found much less frequently (less than 1%). Patients with SLE have a prevalence of 10 to 40% of positive antiphospholipid tests; those with Raynaud's syndrome have a higher incidence of these antibodies. Various infections, malignancies, and drugs can induce antiphospholipid antibodies, but they are thought to be less pathogenic. It has been shown in experimental models that molecular mimicry with infectious agents is possibly involved in the generation of antiphospholipid antibodies and clinical events. Commonly encountered situations of positive antiphospholipid antibodies in humans are listed in **Table 10.1**. Most represent epiphenomena rather than clinically relevant and reproducible findings, except in autoimmune diseases.

In otherwise healthy individuals who have these antibodies, the absolute risk of developing a new thrombosis is less than 1% per year. This risk is considerably higher in patients with associated autoimmune diseases, most notably SLE. In addition, the presence of other risk factors for thromboembolism increases the likelihood of a clinically significant event.

Table 10.1   Conditions Associated with Antiphospholipid Antibodies

DISEASE/CONDITION	EXAMPLES
Autoimmune diseases	Systemic lupus erythematosus, systemic sclerosis, rheumatoid arthritis
Viral infections	HIV, hepatitis C virus, cytomegalovirus, Epstein-Barr virus, parvovirus B19
Bacterial infections	*Streptococcus, Salmonella,* spirochetes (Lyme, syphilis), *Mycoplasma, Coxiella*
Mycobacterial infections	Tuberculosis, leprosy
Malignancies	Leukemia, myeloma, solid tumors
Chronic diseases	Liver disease, chronic renal failure
Medications	Procainamide, hydralazine, quinidine
Healthy subjects	1–10%, age-dependent

The pathogenesis of APS is poorly understood. Antibodies to phospholipids and their binding proteins are a key feature of APS. Multiple mechanisms are thought to contribute to thrombosis and pregnancy-related morbidity. Activation or apoptosis of endothelial cells, platelets, or trophoblasts can induce exposure of phosphatidylserine to the outer surface of cell membranes. Circulating antibodies to β2-glycoprotein I (anti-β2GPI) can consecutively bind to the cell surface and activate the complement cascade. In addition, release of prothrombotic factors propagates the process (e.g., thromboxane from platelets). Furthermore, interference of antiphospholipid antibodies with trophoblast function and annexin V, a placental anticoagulant, can contribute to fetal loss.

CLINICAL AND LABORATORY FEATURES

APS is characterized clinically by recurrent thrombembolic events and pregnancy losses. The original so-called Sapporo criteria to define APS based on clinical and laboratory features have recently been revised and are listed in **Table 10.2**. APS is present if at least one of the clinical criteria and one of the laboratory criteria are met. Positive laboratory results must be obtained on more than one occasion at least 12 weeks apart. Note that classification of APS should not be made if the interval between two positive tests is less than 12 weeks or if more than 5 years separate the positive laboratory test and the clinical manifestation.

Table 10.2   The 2006 Revised Sapporo Criteria for APS[1]

CRITERION	DEFINITION
Clinical criteria	
Vascular thrombosis	One or more clinical episodes of arterial, venous, or small vessel thrombosis, in any tissue or organ. Thrombosis must be confirmed by objective, validated criteria (imaging or histopathology, without significant inflammation in the vessel wall).
Pregnancy morbidity	(a) One or more unexplained deaths of a morphologically normal fetus at or beyond the 10th week of gestation, with normal fetal morphology, *OR* (b) One or more premature births of a morphologically normal neonate before the 34th week of gestation because of: eclampsia or severe preeclampsia, or placental insufficiency, *OR* (c) Three or more unexplained consecutive spontaneous abortions before the 10th week of gestation, with maternal anatomic or hormonal abnormalities and paternal and maternal chromosomal causes excluded.
Laboratory criteria	
Lupus anticoagulant (LA)	LA present in plasma.
Anticardiolipin (aCL)	IgG and/or IgM anticardiolipin antibody isotype, present in medium or high titer (i.e., >40 units, or >99th percentile).
Anti-β2 glycoprotein-I antibody (anti-β2GPI)	Anti-β2GPI of IgG and/or IgM isotype (titer >99th percentile).

Adapted from: Miyakis S, Lockshin MD, Atsumi T, et al. International consensus statement on an update of the classification criteria for definite antiphospholipid syndrome (APS). J. Thromb. Haemost. 2006;4(2):295–306.

Factors such as older age, oral contraceptives, cardiovascular risk factors (including hypertension, diabetes mellitus, hyperlipidemia, obesity, cigarette smoking, and family history of early cardiovascular disease), nephrotic syndrome, cancer, surgery, immobilization, and inherited thrombophilias all contribute to thrombotic risk in the presence of these antibodies.

The two main categories of antiphospolipid antibodies are the anticardiolipin antibodies and the lupus anticoagulant. Anticardiolipin antibodies are assessed by enzyme-linked immunosorbant assay (ELISA). The patient's sera are tested for activity against a cardiolipin-imbedded ELISA plate. The IgG and IgM cardiolipin antibodies are the only isotypes that are accepted as part of the diagnostic criteria. Antibodies directed against beta-2 glycoprotein I can also be used to make the diagnosis. In all cases, the result should be quantified through the use of internationally standardized sera. In addition to anti-β2GPI and anticardiolipin antibodies, antibodies against prothrombin, annexin V, and other antiphospholipids can be detected in APS patients. However, most of these are not yet routinely used because of the lack of standardization. Examples of additional phospholipids targeted in this syndrome include phosphatidylserine, phosphatidylcholin, and phosphatidylethanolamine. A well-known laboratory finding in APS patients is also a false-positive serologic test for syphilis, either the rapid plasma reagin (RPR) or Venereal Disease Research Laboratory (VDRL) tests, due to the presence of cardiolipin in the test reagents. The RPR or VDRL are, however, not recommended for the workup of APS due to their low sensitivity and specificity for this syndrome.

A very important test is the lupus anticoagulant (LA), because it represents a functional assay that is also thought to detect uncharacterized inhibitors. The term lupus anticoagulant can be confusing, because the test is often positive in the absence of SLE (as mentioned earlier; for instance, in primary APS or non-SLE secondary APS). In addition, the putative inhibitors indirectly detected by this assay are considered procoagulants in vivo but act like anticoagulants in vitro, prolonging the activated partial thromboplastin time (aPTT). The discrepancy between the in vitro and in vivo phenomenon is unresolved to date. The exact nature of the LA is also unknown but in some cases may represent anti-β2GPI antibodies that divalently bind phospholipids.

The LA test consists of a mixing study followed by a phospholipid neutralization step. An unexplained prolonged aPTT usually prompts testing for inhibitors or factor deficiencies. In addition, LA testing should be performed if there is a suspicion for primary or secondary APS. The principles of this two-step assay are as follows: first, the patient's plasma is mixed with pooled plasma from normal donors. If an inhibitor (such as LA) is present, the clotting time should be prolonged. A normal aPTT after mixing rules out any inhibitor, including LA, and suggests a factor deficiency. If the mixing study does not correct the clotting time, excess amounts of phospholipids are added to determine if LA is present. If the phospholipids neutralize the suspected lupus anticoagulant, the aPTT should normalize again, which confirms and defines the LA. If the aPTT is still prolonged, it indicates the presence of another inhibitor that does not act via phospholipid binding— that is, LA activity. It is important to note that a positive LA test has a stronger association with thrombosis than do antiphospholipid antibodies measured by ELISA, and the LA test should always be ordered if there is a suspicion for primary or secondary APS.

Vascular Occlusions

Thromboembolic phenomena seen in APS can involve any site of the venous or arterial bed. Venous occlusions have been reported most commonly in the deep veins (with or without associated pulmonary embolism), but also in the renal, mesenteric, portal, and hepatic veins, as well as the inferior vena cava and sagittal sinuses. Arterial sites include the cerebral, retinal, brachial (including its distal branches), mesenteric, and coronary arteries. The clinical manifestations of such occlusions are diverse and depend on the anatomic site. Stroke, bowel ischemia, digital gangrene, or amaurosis fugax are among the various possible presentations. APS is not characterized by significant inflammation in the vessel wall on pathology. If vasculitis is seen, one should consider alternative etiologies.

Obstetric and Neonatal Complications

Obstetric complications include three or more spontaneous abortions prior to week 10 of gestation, a second- or third-trimester intrauterine fetal demise, and preeclampsia. Prematurity, intrauterine growth restriction, and, rarely, neonatal APS due to transplacental passage of IgG anticardiolipin antibodies can also occur.

Hematologic Manifestations

The most common hematologic manifestation is thrombocytopenia. It is rarely clinically significant, but it should be treated like idiopathic thrombocytopenic purpura if symptomatic (e.g., systemic steroids, intravenous immunoglobulin). Autoimmune hemolytic anemia, bone marrow necrosis, and microangiopathies are additional hematologic manifestations reported in APS. Thrombotic thrombocytopenic purpura, hemolytic-uremic syndrome, as well as the HELLP syndrome (hemolysis, elevated liver enzymes, and low platelets during pregnancy) are recognized microangiopathies in APS.

Catastrophic APS

Catastrophic APS is characterized by thrombotic involvement of at least three organs in less than 1 week. Preceding infections or trauma are frequently identified as potential triggers. Intense immunosuppression, cytotoxic agents, and plasmapheresis should be initiated promptly if catastrophic APS is suspected, because mortality exceeds 50%.

Associated Neurologic Syndromes

Various neurologic syndromes other than stroke have also been linked to APS. Cognitive deficits are more frequent in patients with APS, but the causal relationship is currently debated. Weak associations with antiphospholipid antibodies have also been found in patients with migraine, psychosis, recurrent seizures, chorea, sensorineural hearing loss, and transverse myelitis, among others. Magnetic resonance imaging (MRI) of the brain of APS patients can reveal hyperdense central nervous system lesions that are thought to be smaller and nonenhancing compared with those seen in patients suffering from multiple sclerosis. However, this distinction is difficult to make solely based on imaging. It might also be difficult to distinguish clinically, because multiple sclerosis-like and Guillian-Barre syndrome-type signs and symptoms have been associated with APS. Further investigations are necessary to corroborate these associations.

Other Manifestations in APS

Other examples of the diverse clinical features of APS are mitral valve nodules (with associated mitral regurgitation), avascular necrosis of the bones, and cutaneous lesions, such as livedo reticularis, digital necrosis, and splinter hemorrhages. Livedo reticularis in combination with ischemic strokes is called Sneddon syndrome.

Paradoxically, alveolar and adrenal hemorrhage (with consecutive adrenal insufficiency) has also been described in APS patients. Nonthrombotic effects of antiphospholipid antibodies and/or hemorrhagic infarction (e.g., after adrenal vein thrombosis) are potential mechanisms. Finally, a general bleeding diathesis can rarely occur in patients with APS. One should consider investigation of prothrombin inhibitors in these cases, because antibodies to prothrombin are likely responsible for this peculiar phenomenon.

MANAGEMENT

Prophylactic Measures in Individuals with Positive Antiphospholipid Antibodies

The clinical significance of positive antiphospholipid antibodies or a lupus anticoagulant in otherwise healthy individuals is unclear. Pharmacologic therapy is not necessary in this situation. A recent randomized, double-blind, placebo-controlled trial demonstrated no benefit from even low-dose aspirin in asymptomatic patients with persistently positive antiphospholipid antibodies for primary thrombosis prophylaxis. These patients had a low overall annual incidence rate of acute thrombosis without additional risk factors for thrombosis.

However, nonpharmacologic measures are certainly useful for primary prevention in this population. General counseling, as with patients with thromboembolic events due to other causes, includes smoking cessation, weight loss, and an active lifestyle, if not already pursued. Estrogen-containing contraceptives (including oral, ring, or patch formulations) are contraindicated in patients with APS and should not be used in asymptomatic patients with positive antiphospholipid antibodies. Progesterone-only products and barrier methods are possible alternatives.

Warfarin Treatment

Lifelong anticoagulation is necessary in most APS patients with thrombosis, but it carries significant risks for bleeding complications. A randomized, double-blind trial compared warfarin at moderate intensity (INR between 2 to 3) versus high intensity (INR between 3 and 4) for this patient population. Based on this trial and other recent studies, an INR target of 2 to 3 is likely sufficient to prevent future events. This regimen can at least be recommended in patients who are not at highest risk or who do not present with predominantly arterial, noncerebral clots. These patients might still benefit from the traditional anticoagulation target of an INR between 3 and 4. In general, the optimal treatment for APS patients with thromboembolic events still needs to be assessed on an individual basis; additional risk factors for such events as well as contraindications to anticoagulation therapy must be taken into account.

Treatment of APS Patients During Pregnancy

Warfarin is absolutely contraindicated during pregnancy due to its teratogenic potential. Low-molecular-weight heparin can be safely used in pregnant patients. It is the preferred option during pregnancy because it offers better bioavailability, fewer injections, and better safety regarding heparin-induced thrombocytopenia and osteoporosis compared with unfractionated heparin.

Only a few studies are available regarding the treatment of APS patients during pregnancy. Most recommendations are based on expert opinions. Patients with APS due to obstetric complications alone should be treated with low-dose aspirin and prophylactic-dose low-molecular-weight heparin (or unfractionated heparin) and kept on low-dose aspirin indefinitely after delivery. APS patients with previous thrombosis need to be treated with therapeutic dose heparin products and low-dose aspirin. Addition of intravenous immunoglobulins to aspirin and heparin can be considered during pregnancy in refractory cases.

Other Treatment Options

In addition to aspirin, heparin products, and warfarin, other agents have been used in APS patients. Scarce data is available for antiplatelet agents such as dipyridamole, clopidogrel, or ticlopidine. Treatment with the antimalarial drug hydroxychloroquine has been associated with reduced risk of thrombosis in experimental models of APS. It is also a well-tolerated and effective therapy in mild lupus, as discussed in the chapter on SLE, and reduces thrombotic events in this patient population. Hydroxychloroquine has been shown to directly reduce the binding of antiphospholipid antibody–β2-glycoprotein I complexes to phospholipid bilayers. Prospective clinical trials are needed to confirm the efficacy of hydroxychloroquine for APS.

Finally, patients who have failed warfarin therapy can be tried on thrombin inhibitors (e.g., argatroban) or rituximab, a monoclonal antibody directed against B cells (targeting CD20). Novel therapies include attempts to tolerize pathogenic B cells, inhibit the complement cascade, or block certain cytokines. The anti-inflammatory and antithrombotic effects of statins are theoretically also beneficial in APS, but have not yet been formally studied.

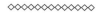

REFERENCES

1.   Miyakis S, Lockshin MD, Atsumi T, et al. International consensus statement on an update of the classification criteria for definite antiphospholipid syndrome (APS). *J. Thromb. Haemost.* 2006;4(2): 295–306.

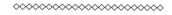

SUGGESTED READINGS

Crowther MA, Ginsberg JS, Julian J, et al. A comparison of two intensities of warfarin for the prevention of recurrent thrombosis in patients with the antiphospholipid antibody syndrome. *N Engl J. Med.* 2003;349:1133–1138.

Firestein GS, Budd RC, Harris ED Jr., McInnis IB, Ruddy S, Sergent JS. *Kelley's textbook of rheumatology,* 8th ed. New York: Elsevier Saunders; 2009.

Greer JP, Foerster J, Rodgers GM, et al. *Wintrobe's clinical hematology,* 12th ed. Philadelphia: Wolters Kluwer Health/Lippincott Williams & Wilkins; 2009.

Hochberg MC, Silman AJ, Smolen JS, Weinblatt ME, Weisman MH. *Rheumatology,* 4th ed. New York: Elsevier; 2009.

Lahita RG. *Systemic lupus erythematosus,* 4th ed. New York: Elsevier, Academic Press; 2004.

Lim W, Crowther MA, Eikelboom JW. Management of antiphospholipid antibody syndrome: a systematic review. *JAMA.* 2006;295:1050–1057.

Tsokos GC, Gordon PC, Smolen JS (eds.). *Systemic lupus erythematosus: a companion to rheumatology.* New York: Elsevier; 2007.

Wallace DJ. *Lupus: the essential clinician's guide.* New York: Oxford University Press; 2008.

Wallace DJ, Hahn BH. *Dubois' lupus erythematosus,* 7th ed. Philadelphia: Lippencott Williams and Wilkins; 2006.

CHAPTER 11

Approach to Vasculitides

Kichul Shin MD, PhD

OVERVIEW

Vasculitides comprise a heterogeneous group of localized or systemic diseases that share the clinical characteristic of vessel wall inflammation. Constitutional symptoms of fever or weight loss, arthralgia, myalgia, and skin rashes are some of the many clinical manifestations of vasculitic disorders. Differential diagnoses include infection, drug-induced or thrombotic disorders, and malignancy. Several classification systems for vasculitis are available; some are based on the size of the vessels involved and others are based on the extent of the disease (**Tables 11.1** and **11.2**). For the purpose of this chapter, we will use the system based on vessel size.

Table 11.1 Classification of Vasculitides (I)[1]

DOMINANT VESSEL	TYPE OF VASCULITIS
Large-sized arteries	Giant cell arteritis Takayasu's arteritis Primary angiitis of the central nervous system
Medium-sized arteries	Polyarteritis nodosa Kawasaki disease
Small vessels and medium-sized arteries	Wegener's granulomatosis Churg-Strauss syndrome Microscopic polyangiitis
Small-sized vessels	Henoch-Schönlein purpura Cryoglobulinemia Leukocytoclastic vasculitis

Jennette, J.C., et al., Nomenclature of systemic vasculitides. Proposal of an international consensus conference. Arthritis Rheum. 1994. 37(2): p. 187-92.

Diagnosis of vasculitis is based on clinical features, the extent and type of vessel involvement, laboratory testing, organ or vessel imaging, and tissue biopsy. Treatment can range from no medication to significant use of immunosuppressive and cytotoxic agents.

Table 11.2 Classification of Vasculitides (II)[2]

I. Systemic necrotizing vasculitis
   A. Polyarteritis nodosa (PAN)
      1. Classic PAN
      2. Microscopic polyangiitis
   B. Churg-Strauss syndrome
   C. Polyangiitis overlap syndrome
II. Wegener's granulomatosis
III. Temporal arteritis
IV. Takayasu's arteritis
V. Henoch-Schönlein purpura
VI. Predominantly cutaneous vasculitis (hypersensitivity vasculitis)
   A. Exogenous stimuli proven or suspected
      1. Drug-induced vasculitis
      2. Serum sickness and serum sickness-like reactions
      3. Vasculitis associated with infectious diseases
   B. Endogenous antigens likely involved
      1. Vasculitis associated with connective tissue diseases
      2. Vasculitis associated with other underlying diseases
      3. Vasculitis associated with congenital deficiencies of the complement system
VII. Other vasculitic syndromes
   A. Kawasaki disease
   B. Isolated central nervous system vasculitis
   C. Thromboangiitis obliterans (Buerger's disease)
   D. Behcet's syndrome
   E. Miscellaneous vasculitides

Adapted from Sneller MC, Fauci AS. Pathogenesis of vasculitis syndromes. Med Clin North Am. 1997;81(10):221-42

CLASSIFICATION

Clinical Manifestations

Vasculitides often present with systemic symptoms such as fevers, weight loss, malaise, anemia, and hypoalbumimia. Specific symptoms are related to the size of the vessel involved (**Table 11.3**).

Table 11.3   Clinical Features of Vasculitis on the Basis of Size of the Affected Blood Vessel[3]

SIZE OF BLOOD VESSEL	BLOOD VESSEL INVOLVED	CLINICAL FEATURES
Large	Extracranial branches of carotid artery	Temporal headache (temporal artery), blindness (ophthalmic artery), jaw claudication (vessels supplying vessels of mastication)
	Thoracic aorta and its branches	Limb claudication, absent pulses and unequal blood pressure, bruits, thoracic aortic aneurysm
Medium	Small cutaneous arteries	Necrotic lesions and ulcers, nail fold infarcts
	Vasa nervorum	Mononeuritis multiplex
	Mesenteric artery	Abdominal pain, gastrointestinal bleeding, perforation
	Branches of celiac artery	Infarction of liver, spleen, pancreas
	Renal artery	Renal infarction
	Coronary arteries	Myocardial infarction or angina, coronary artery aneurysm, ischemic cardiomyopathy
	Small pulmonary arteries	Necrotic lesions leading to cavitating lung shadows on chest radiograph
	Small arteries in ear, nose, throat	Nasal crusting, epistaxis, sinusitis, deafness, stridor
Small	Cutaneous postcapillary venules	Palpable purpura
	Glomerular capillaries	Hematuria, red cell casts in urine, proteinuria, decline in renal function
	Pulmonary capillaries	Lung hemorrhage manifesting as shortness of breath, hemoptysis, alvelolar shadowing on chest radiograph

Suresh, E. Diagnostic approach to patients with suspected vasculitis. Postgrad Med. J. 2006;82(970):483–488.

Differential Diagnosis

Infections, in particular syphilis, tuberculosis, human immunodeficiency virus (HIV), and endocarditis can present with features similar to vasculitides. Malignancies, especially hematologic malignancies, can be difficult to distinguish from vasculitides.

DIAGNOSTIC INVESTIGATIONS

A careful clinical history should be obtained, including ingestion history of drugs, presence of preexisting symptoms suggestive of acute or chronic systemic disorders, autoimmune diseases, and a history of recent or chronic infection. This should be followed by a thorough physical examination. **Table 11.4** outlines investigations to consider during the initial evaluation of patients with suspected vasculitis.

Table 11.4   Investigations to Consider During Initial Evaluation of Patients with Suspected Vasculitis

To exclude vasculitis mimics and secondary causes:

Blood cultures, ECG, antiphospholipid antibodies
Hepatitis B and C screen, HIV test, antinuclear antibodies, anti-double strand DNA antibody

To assess specific type of vasculitis:

Antineutrophil cytoplasmic antibody (ANCA), cryoglobulin, complement levels, eosinophil count, IgE levels

To confirm the diagnosis of vasculitis:

Biopsy and/or angiography

To assess extent of vasculitis:

Urinalysis
Chest radiography
Nerve conduction study, electromyography, creatine kinase

Laboratory Tests

Laboratory tests should test for secondary causes or etiologies, such as the following:

- Infections: hepatitis B and C serologies, anti-HIV
- Autoimmune disorders: antinuclear antibody, anti-double strand DNA antibody
- Immune complex disorders: complement levels (C3,C4), cryoglobulin

Disease-specific laboratory testing includes testing for antineutrophil cytoplasmic antibody (ANCA), which is found in the serum of patients with specific types of vasculitis. It is normally measured by indirect immunofluorescence (IF) and enzyme-linked immunosorbent assay (ELISA). Two different staining patterns are cytoplasmic [c-ANCA, reflecting antibodies to serine protease 3 (PR3)] and perinuclear [p-ANCA, reacting to myeloperoxidase (MPO)]. The combination of positive c-ANCA and anti-PR3 is strongly associated with Wegener's granulomatosis (WG). The p-ANCA pattern and anti-MPO occurs in about 10% of WG, but is more typical of microscopic polyangiitis, or Churg-Strauss syndrome. In the setting of active vasculitis, 10% of WG patients may be negative for ANCA. Therefore, the definite diagnosis of vasculitis should be based on clinical signs and tissue biopsy results, not on ANCA positivity. In general, ANCA titers have imperfect correlations with disease activity.

Organ-specific laboratory testing should include routine blood testing, erythrocyte sedimentation rate (ESR), and C-reactive protein (CRP). Specifically, renal involvement can be evaluated by measurement of serum creatinine, urinalysis, urine sediment assessment, and 24-hour urine collection for determination of creatinine clearance and protein. Muscle damage resulting from inflammation can be reflected in elevated creatinine kinase or aldolase levels. Elevated liver function tests may also suggest occult muscle involvement. Abnormal results of liver function tests may reflect liver inflammation or associated infectious hepatitis. The cerebrospinal fluid (CSF) is analyzed to check cell count, differential count, and chemistry in addition to investigations to rule out infectious diseases.

Imaging Studies

Imaging studies may include plain radiograph (e.g., posteroanterior and lateral chest radiograph or sinus series), ultrasonography, computed tomography (CT) and magnetic resonance imaging (MRI), angiography, or positron-emission tomography (PET).

The use of ultrasonography (US) is mostly limited to assessment of large vessels. Temporal artery US can be used to guide the surgeon to the artery segment with the clearest "halo" sign representing edema to perform a biopsy.[4] The distal subclavian, axillary, and brachial arteries can also be examined by US.

CT and MRI can be used to help determine the presence of specific organ involvement or extent of disease, such as chest CT to evaluate lung disease or brain MRI to assess infarcts.

Angiography can provide diagnostic accuracy and definition of the type and extent of vascular involvement. Conventional percutaneous transcatheter angiography is the gold standard of angiography. Magnetic resonance angiography (MRA) can be employed as a noninvasive method of evaluating vessel involvement. Angiography should be performed judiciously in patients with renal function impairment, especially when using gadolinium containing contrast agents in patients with a glomerular filtration rate (GFR) less than 30 mL/min/$1.73m^2$ to prevent nephrogenic systemic fibrosis.[5]

PET can be used in select cases for showing aortic and other vascular inflammation as part of the diagnostic workup.

Histologic Assessment

A tissue biopsy should be considered in cases with an undefined diagnosis, to guide further therapy, or to clarify the prognosis.

OVERVIEW OF RESPECTIVE DISEASES

Giant Cell Arteritis

Giant cell arteritis (GCA) is a disease of aging adults; onset is usually after the age of 50. It primarily affects Caucasians, and women are twice as likely as men to be affected. GCA can accompany polymyalgia rheumatica (PMR).

Presenting symptoms include fatigue, headache, jaw claudication (pain with chewing), and tenderness of the scalp, particularly around the temporal and occipital areas. Half of the patients have proximal soreness and joint symptoms of PMR. Sometimes the ascending aorta and/or aortic arch and its branches are involved.

Upon physical examination, the temporal arteries can be tender, palpable, and nodular with reduced pulsation. Transient visual impairment can lead to permanent blindness if not treated promptly.

A diagnosis of GCA should be considered in any patient older than 50 years with recent onset of headache, loss of vision, myalgia, high ESR, anemia, or sometimes fever of unknown origin. Laboratory results will show an ESR usually elevated above 100 mm/h, but a normal ESR does not rule out GCA. Normocytic normochromic anemia and thrombocytosis are common.

A temporal artery biopsy is an important diagnostic procedure to confirm the diagnosis. Bilateral temporal artery biopsy is performed, considering false negatives in case of skipped lesions. Pathology shows granulomatous arteritis with giant cells and destruction of the internal elastic lamina. If clinical suspicion is high and the initial biopsy is negative, a biopsy of the contralateral temporal artery should be performed. Note that treatment should not be delayed while awaiting biopsy results.

Treatment generally includes starting high dose (40 to 60 mg) of prednisone; tapering by roughly 10mg/day each month normally begins after a month. Patients will usually need to be on steroids for about a year or more. Patients should be aware of the side effects of corticosteroids, and preventive measures against steroid-induced osteoporosis should be considered upfront. Low-dose aspirin (100 mg) has been shown to prevent ischemic complications of GCA.[6]

Takayasu's Arteritis

Takayasu's arteritis (TA) is a chronic inflammatory disorder of unknown etiology that affects the aorta and its major branches. It predominantly affects women between the ages of 15 to 25. Clinical manifestations include malaise, fever, night sweats, weight loss, myalgia, symptoms of claudication, headaches, syncope, and visual disturbances. Upon physical examination, patients will elicit a weak or even absent pulse in the upper extremities or arterial bruits over the involved vessels. Hypertension is common.

Diagnosis of TA should be considered when symptoms of vascular insufficiency (claudication, transient visual disturbances, syncope) occur in the setting of bruits, weak pulses, and discrepancies of four-limb blood pressure in young women with constitutional symptoms. Laboratory findings include anemia and thrombocytosis. ESR and CRP could be elevated, but these markers are often normal and do not directly correlate with disease activity. Conventional or MR angiography demonstrates a segmental, smooth, tapered pattern of stenosis or complete occlusion of a large vessel. Visualization of the whole aorta is needed.

The mainstay treatment is oral corticosteroids. Most patients respond to a dosage of 1 mg/kg/day; alternatively, a starting dose of 30 mg/day with a maintenance dose of 5 to 10 mg/day is effective. Low-dose aspirin or other antiplatelet agents should complement corticosteroid therapy. Cytotoxic therapy has been used in patients failing steroid treatment. Vascular surgery and percutaneous transluminal angioplasty have also been used in cases of advanced disease, with variable success.

Primary Angiitis of the CNS

Primary angiitis is a rare vasculitic disorder localized to the CNS. Common clinical symptoms include headache, which can spontaneously remit for long periods. Non-focal neurologic deficits are characteristic, such as decrease in cognitive function. Depending on the anatomic area or disease extent, features may range from transient ischemic attack, strokes, cranial neuropathies, to seizures.

CSF analysis may reflect pleocytosis, normal glucose levels, and increased protein. CSF should also be assessed for possibilities of infection. MRI and CT provide suggestive findings, including multiple, bilateral brain infarcts. Angiography has proven to be less useful in this case. Histologic confirmation is supported by a leptomeningeal biopsy demonstrating granulomatous vasculitis.[7]

Treatment includes high-dose corticosteroids (1 mg/kg/day) or cytotoxic agents, such as cyclophosphamide.

Polyarteritis Nodosa

Polyarteritis nodosa (PAN) is a necrotizing vasculitis of medium-sized and small arteries. The etiology of PAN is mostly unknown, but viruses, including hepatitis B virus, HIV, cytomegalovirus, parvovirus B19, human T lymphotrophic virus type 1, and hepatitis C virus, have been implicated as etiologic agents.

Patients present with constitutional symptoms, such as malaise, fever, and weight loss; cutaneous or gastrointestinal involvement; and peripheral neuropathy. Cutaneous lesions are present in about 50% of patients. The lesions are typically papulo-petechial. Livedo reticularis is common. Gastrointestinal manifestations can be severe, presenting with abdominal pain, bleeding, or bowel perforation. Painful mononeuritis multiplex or mononeuropathies manifested by dropped foot or hand may be seen. Kidney involvement is related to vascular compromise but not glomerulonephritis. Testicular involvement occurs in over 25% of men with this disorder. Diagnostic criteria for PAN are provided in **Table 11.5**. At least three criteria must be present for a diagnosis of PAN.

Table 11.5   American College of Rheumatology Criteria Diagnosis of PAN[12]

AT LEAST **3** OF **10** CRITERIA:
1. Weight loss ≥4 kg
2. Livedo reticularis
3. Testicular pain or tenderness
4. Myalgias, weakness, or leg tenderness
5. Mononeuropathy or polyneuropathy
6. Diastolic blood pressure >90 mm Hg
7. Elevated serum nitrogen urea (>40 mg/dL) or creatinine (>1.5 mg/dL)
8. Hepatitis B virus infection
9. Arteriographic abnormality
10. Biopsy of small- or medium-sized artery containing polymorphonuclear neutrophils

Reprinted with permission from John Wiley & Sons, Inc.

Laboratory results may reflect leukocytosis and thrombocytosis, and the ESR and CRP are usually high. PAN is not associated with ANCA. Hepatitis B surface antigen should be checked in all cases.

Angiographic findings include lesions of microaneurysms and stenosis/poststenotic dilation of medium-sized vessels.

Candidate tissue sites for biopsy include the skin, skeletal muscle, sural nerve, and kidney, depending on the clinical features. Skin biopsy specimen should include the sub-dermis to detect medium-sized vessel involvement. The pathology seen in PAN is a focal, segmental, necrotizing vasculitis of medium-sized and small vessels. Arterial aneurysms and thromboses can occur at the site of the vascular lesion.

In hepatitis B-related PAN, antiviral agents accompanied by plasma exchange and short courses of corticosteroids are helpful. In the absence of hepatitis B involvement, high doses of corticosteroids are used for initial management. Cyclophosphamide is added for severe cases as an induction therapy followed by azathioprine.

Kawasaki Disease

Kawasaki disease is an acute febrile disease occurring mostly in infants and children younger than 5 years. Onset is typically abrupt, with remitting or continuous high fever that generally lasts 1 to 2 weeks. Within 4 days of onset, bilateral conjunctival injection occurs with dryness, redness, and fissuring of the lips as well as a "strawberry" tongue.

Painful cervical lymphadenopathy appears with the fever. Exanthema of the trunk and redness of palms and soles are seen, resulting in desquamation. Other symptoms include abdominal pain, vomiting, diarrhea, and arthritis. Vasculitis is most commonly seen in the medium-sized and large arteries, including the coronary and iliac arteries. Coronary vasculitis is the most serious and life-threatening complication; sometimes lesions can be shown by dilatation or aneurysms in ECG. Other cardiovascular involvement includes carditis with heart murmurs and ECG changes.

Differential diagnoses of acute febrile illnesses with rash such as measles, scarlet fever, viral exanthems, and drug reactions should be assessed.

Uncomplicated cases are based on supportive management. Coronary artery involvement should be checked by ECG weekly for a month. If changes are detected, an infusion of high-dose intravenous gamma-globulin (2 g/kg) is given. Low-dose aspirin is used until the coronary artery changes regress.

Wegener's Granulomatosis

The classic triad of Wegener's granulomatosis (WG) is necrotizing granulomatous vasculitis of the upper and lower airways, systemic vasculitis, and focal necrotizing glomerulonephritis. A subset of "limited" WG is a milder and less aggressive disease that involves the airways in the absence of glomerulonephritis. WG similarly affects male and female.

Most WG patients have upper and lower respiratory tract symptoms, commonly with sinus pain, discharge, nasal mucosa ulceration, otitis media, and tracheal inflammation. Alveolar capillaritis can cause pulmonary hemorrhage leading to hemoptysis, hypoxemia, and anemia. Pulmonary or renal problems, or both, eventually develop in more than 80% of patients. Other features include ocular inflammation, cutaneous purpura, peripheral neuropathy, arthritis, and diverse abdominal visceral involvement.

Laboratory tests show normocytic normochromic anemia, leukocytosis, thrombocytosis, and elevated ESR and CRP. ANCA, especially c-ANCA, is associated with WG. It has high specificity (~98%) yet lower sensitivity. Elevated titers usually reflect active disease; however c-ANCA titer itself does not strongly correlate with disease activity. Five percent of patients can be p-ANCA positive. Chest radiograph and CT demonstrate pulmonary infiltrates or nodules. The strongest evidence comes from biopsy results showing granulomas. In renal biopsies, focal necrosis and crescent formation in the glomeruli, as well as absence of immunoglobulin deposits (pauci-immune), may be identified.

Treatment includes high doses of intravenous and oral corticosteroids plus cyclophosphamide for induction therapy. Pulse intravenous and oral (2 mg/kg/day) cyclophosphamide are equally effective in achieving initial remission. Oral cyclophosphamide is superior to the pulse intravenous regimen in preventing relapses of WG. Cyclophosphamide dose adjustment is monitored by blood leukocyte counts. Trimethoprim/sulfamethoxazole is normally added not only to prevent *Pneumocystis carinii* infection, but also to help WG treatment itself. Prednisone is gradually tapered off, and cyclophosphamide is switched to methotrexate or azathioprine after 6 months for maintenance therapy.

Microscopic Polyangiitis

Microscopic polyangiitis (MPA) is a pauci-immune necrotizing vasculitis without evidence of granulomatous inflammation. Patients present with an insidious onset of pulmonary-renal syndrome, predominantly having glomerulonephritis.

Most patients are p-ANCA positive. Pathologically, MPA and PAN can be indistinguishable. The two entities can be differentiated by the absence of vasculitis in vessels other than the arteries in PAN and the presence of vasculitis in vessels smaller than arteries by MPA.

Corticosteroids and cytotoxic agents are the mainstay of treatment, similar to the treatment of WG. About one-third of patients relapse and are retreated with a regimen similar to the induction therapy.

Churg-Strauss Syndrome

Churg-Strauss syndrome (CSS) is a form of vasculitis occurring in individuals with asthma and allergic rhinitis. It features inflammation of blood vessels (also referred to as angiitis) in the lungs, skin, nerves, and abdomen.

Pulmonary infiltrates, cutaneous eruptions, and peripheral neuropathy are common clinical features. Cardiac involvement, such as pericarditis, cardiomyopathy, and myocardial infarction, could lead to critical outcomes. Renal disease is rare and generally mild.

Laboratory findings show ANCA positivity in 70% of patients, mainly p-ANCA, as well as anemia, elevated ESR, and peripheral eosinophilia. In addition to tissue eosinophilia, the presence of vasculitis and granulomas can help differentiate CSS from chronic eosinophilic pneumonia and idiopathic hypereosinophilic syndrome. The biopsy result and the association with allergic disease can help differentiate CSS from other ANCA-positive vasculitides.

Initial management consists of high-dose corticosteroids such as prednisone (1 mg/kg/day). Life-threatening complications require the addition of cyclophosphamide or azathioprine. Relapses are rare after complete remission.

Henoch-Schönlein Purpura

Henoch-Schönlein purpura (HSP) is the most common vasculitis occurring during childhood, with a self-limited course in most patients.

The classic triad is palpable purpura with normal platelet count, colicky abdominal pain, and arthritis. Palpable purpura occurs in the dependent areas, especially the buttocks. Half of patients have occult gastrointestinal bleeding, but serious hemorrhages are rare. Renal involvement, ranging from microscopic hematuria to rapidly progressive glomerulonephritis, occurs in 10 to 50% of patients. Adult-onset HSP tends to have a higher incidence of severe renal manifestations.

Diagnosis is based on clinical features, and laboratory findings are used to assess the extent of the disease. IgA deposits are appreciated in skin or kidney biopsies.

Treatment is primarily supportive management. Corticosteroids have been used in the treatment of abdominal pain, edema, and nephritis. Cyclophosphamide is considered in severe kidney involvement.

Cryoglobulinemia

Cryoglobulins are circulating immunoglobulins that precipitate at low temperatures. Type 1 cryoglobulinemia is composed of single monoclonal IgG or IgM. Type 2 is composed of a monoclonal component with activity toward polyclonal immunoglobulins. Type 3 is composed of two or more polyclonal immunoglobulins. Mixed (type 2 and 3) cryoglobulinemia leads to immune complex disease by depositing in the vessels and activating complement, which results in inflammation. Hepatitis C virus infection is one of the important etiologies of mixed cryoglobulinemia.

The most common clinical manifestations are palpable purpura, arthralgia, and nephritis. Furthermore, Raynaud's phenomenon, skin ulcers, and splenomegaly can also be found.

To detect cryoglobulin in serum, blood must be maintained at 37°C during transport and clotting, followed by serum storage at 4°C for at least 7 days. Cryocrit measures the percentage of packed cryoglobulins in serum after centrifugation. Cryocrit may be up to 50% in type 1 cryoglobulinemia. No correlation exists between the cryocrit and disease severity. Rheumatoid factor could be detected in the serum as well as very low C4 levels. Skin biopsy shows findings of leukocytoclastic vasculitis.

Mild disease with arthralgia and purpura is usually treated with nonsteroidal anti-inflammatory drugs (NSAIDs). Interferon-α is used in cryoglobulinemic vasculitis with hepatitis C virus infection. Options for severe clinical manifestations, such as glomerulonephritis, include corticosteroids, plasmapheresis, and rituximab.

Leukocytoclastic Vasculitis

Leukocytoclastic vasculitis (LV) is also known as *hypersensitivity vasculitis*. Etiologies include drugs (e.g., allopurinol), infection (e.g., lyme disease, viral exanthema), malignancies, and idiopathic LV. LV could be also seen in RA, SLE, Sjogren's syndrome, and other vasculitides.

Skin shows nonblanching palpable purpura, mostly in dependent areas, which usually resolves in 1 to 2 weeks. Systemic signs may include fever, arthritis, headaches, pericarditis, and nephritis.

Laboratory tests are performed to rule out other disease entities. Biopsy of lesions demonstrates nonspecific vascular inflammation, infiltration of neutrophils, sometimes with cell destruction, and liberating nuclear dust (leukocytoclasis).

Potential precipitating agents should be discontinued and avoided in the future. For mild skin-limited disease, colchicine or dapsone may be used. In severe cases, steroids and immunosuppressive agents may be used and tapered slowly.

Behcet's Disease

Behcet's disease is a systemic vasculitis involving both arteries and veins. It is mainly observed in people of Mediterranean and Asian descent.

The clinical manifestation is characterized by a syndrome of recurrent, discrete painful oral and genital aphthous ulcers, uveitis, nonspecific hyperreactivity of skin (pathergy reaction), erythema nodosum, and superficial thrombophlebitis. CNS involvement is rare, but has been observed. Symptoms and signs fluctuate with time.

No laboratory test is available for diagnosis. Diagnosis is made by a skin pathergy test (skin is pricked with a sterile 20-gauge needle and followed for 48 hours to see if an erythematous papule or pustule forms at the puncture site) that can be performed on the forearm or back.

Colchicine is effective mainly for mucocutaneous lesions. Local corticosteroids or thalidomide is also helpful. For uveitis, short-term use of steroids is utilized followed by immunosuppressive agents, such as azathioprine or cyclosporine A.

SECONDARY CAUSES

Infections often coexist with vasculitis, especially infections such as hepatitis B and C, HIV, infective endocarditis, and tuberculosis. Any underlying infectious etiology should be treated upfront before starting immunosuppressive therapy. For instance, PAN secondary to hepatitis B should be first treated with antiviral drugs, not cyclophosphamide. Vasculitis could associate with connective tissue disease, including RA, Sjogren's syndrome, SLE, and relapsing polychondritis. Common clinical manifestations of rheumatoid vasculitis include fever, weight loss, digital ischemia, skin purpura or ulcers, and mononeuritis multiplex. Cutaneous presentations of primary Sjogren's syndrome include cryoglobulinemia vasculitis, urticarial vasculitis, and cutaneous purpura unassociated with cryoglobulins.[8] Drug-induced vasculitis could induce a wide range of manifestations, from isolated cutaneous vasculitis to widespread internal organ involvement. Drugs such as hydralazine, propylthiouracil, and monelukast have been implicated in ANCA-associated (preferably p-ANCA) vasculitis.[9,10] Resolution of vasculitis is likely to occur after withdrawal of offending agent. Other secondary causes include inflammatory bowel disease, sarcoidosis, and solid and hematologic malignancies.

SINGLE-ORGAN VASCULITIS

Single-organ vasculitis is usually an unexpected finding in resected tissues affecting abdominal and genitourinary organs, breasts, and the aorta.[11] Patients may present with focal inflammatory or noninflammatory abnormalities. Many of these cases may be cured with resection of the involved tissues, and some may regress spontaneously. Systemic immunosuppressive therapy is usually not required. Definitive diagnosis of single-organ vasculitis requires careful initial assessment to exclude systemic involvement and long-term surveillance to confirm the absence of systemic disease.

SUMMARY

The approach to diagnosing suspected vasculitides is to start by ruling out the mimickers of vasculitis such as infectious diseases, drug-induced or thrombotic disorders, and malignancies. However, sometimes infection (e.g., hepatitis B) or a drug (e.g., hydralazine) can be associated with vasculitis. After a careful history and physical exam, it is helpful to try to characterize the involved vessels' size (small, medium, or large). This, in conjunction with laboratory tests, imaging studies, and histologic assessment are important tools to make the final diagnosis.

◇◇◇◇◇◇◇◇◇◇◇◇

REFERENCES

1. Jennette JC, Falk RJ, Andrassy K, et al. Nomenclature of systemic vasculitides. Proposal of an international consensus conference. *Arthritis Rheum.* 1994;37(2):187–192.

2. Kasper DL, Fauci AS, Longo DL, Braunwald E, Hauser SL, Jameson JL, eds. *Harrison's Principles of Internal Medicine.* 15th ed. Table 317-1. New York, NY: McGraw-Hill; 2001.

3. Suresh E. Diagnostic approach to patients with suspected vasculitis. *Postgrad Med J.* 2006;82(970):483–488.

4. Blockmans D, Bley T, Schmidt W. Imaging for large-vessel vasculitis. *Curr Opin Rheumatol.* 2009;21(1):19–28.

5. Kay J. Nephrogenic systemic fibrosis: a new concern for rheumatologists. *Nat Clin Pract Rheumatol.* 2008;4(9):445.

6. Nesher G, Berkun Y, Mates M, Baras M, Robinow A, Sonnenblick M. Low-dose aspirin and prevention of cranial ischemic complications in giant cell arteritis. *Arthritis Rheum.* 2004;50(4):1332–1337.

7. Calabrese LH, Mallek JA. Primary angiitis of the central nervous system. Report of 8 new cases, review of the literature, and proposal for diagnostic criteria. *Medicine (Baltimore).* 1988;67(1):20–39.

8. Ramos-Casals M, Anaya JM, Garcia-Carrasco M, et al. Cutaneous vasculitis in primary Sjogren syndrome: classification and clinical significance of 52 patients. *Medicine (Baltimore).* 2004;83(2):96–106.

9. Choi HK, Slot MC, Pan G, Weissbach CA, Niles JL, Merhel PA. Evaluation of antineutrophil cytoplasmic antibody seroconversion induced by minocycline, sulfasalazine, or penicillamine. *Arthritis Rheum.* 2000;43(11):2488–2492.

10. Bonaci-Nikolic B, Nikolic MM, Andrejevic S, Zoric S, Bukilica M. Antineutrophil cytoplasmic antibody (ANCA)-associated autoimmune diseases induced by antithyroid drugs: comparison with idiopathic ANCA vasculitides. *Arthritis Res Ther.* 2005;7(5):R1072–R1081.

11. Hernandez-Rodriguez J, Molloy ES, Hoffman GS. Single-organ vasculitis. *Curr Opin Rheumatol.* 2008;20(1):40–46.

12. Lightfoot RW, Michel BA, Block DA, et al. The American College of Rheumatology 1990 Criteria for the classification of polyarteritis nodosa. *Arteritis Rheum.* 1990;33:1088–1093.

CHAPTER 12

Crystal-Induced Arthropathies

Joerg Ermann, MD

OVERVIEW

This chapter discusses arthropathies that occur secondary to local crystal deposition. In particular, gout caused by monosodium uric acid crystals and pseudogout caused by calcium pyrophosphate dihydrate (CPPD) will be reviewed in detail, with shorter discussions of other crystal-induced arthropathies.

GOUT

Gout is the most common crystal-induced arthropathy. Gout occurs in the setting of hyperuricemia (serum uric acid >6.4 mg/dL) and is caused by the deposition of uric acid monosodium crystals in or around joints. It is helpful to distinguish between four clinical stages: asymptomatic hyperuricemia, acute gout, intercritical gout, and chronic tophaceous gout.

Asymptomatic Hyperuricemia

Uric acid is the end product of purine catabolism in humans (**Figure 12.1**). In contrast to most other mammals, humans lack the enzyme uricase, which degrades uric acid. Therefore, even healthy normal humans may have serum uric acid levels close to the saturation point (6.8 mg/dL) above which crystals can form. Uric acid is excreted mainly through the kidneys. Primary hyperuricemia is common and its prevalence increases with age. Estrogen appears to be protective for the development of hyperuricemia; it is rare to see hyperuricemia or gout in premenopausal women. In the vast majority of cases, hyperuricemia is caused by reduced renal excretion. Metabolic defects leading to increased production of uric acid are much less common. Secondary hyperuricemia can occur as a result of increased cell turnover (hematologic malignancies, tumor lysis syndrome, psoriasis), chronic kidney disease, or drugs that interfere with uric acid excretion (e.g., cyclosporine, diuretics). Hyperuricemia is also a component of the metabolic syndrome. Whether an elevated serum uric acid level constitutes an independent risk factor for cardiovascular disease is under investigation.[1] Only a fraction of individuals with hyperuricemia will develop gouty arthritis.

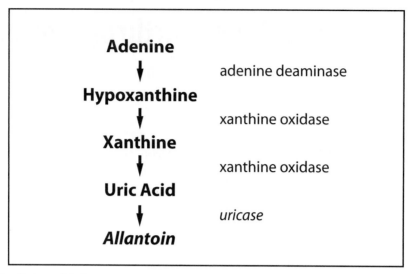

Figure 12.1   Purine metabolism

Acute Gout

The risk for gout increases with the degree of hyperuricemia. Why it occurs only sporadically and in some individuals with hyperuricemia is poorly understood. Once uric acid crystals are formed, they can activate innate immune cells through the inflammasome, a cytoplasmic structure that activates the highly proinflammatory cytokine interleukin-1. Several factors can trigger an acute gout attack: trauma, surgery, starvation, dietary excess, alcohol consumption (in particular beer and spirits), and initiation or discontinuation of uric acid-lowering drugs.

The typical gout attack is an acute monoarthritis. It is characterized by severe pain, erythema, and swelling. The most commonly affected joint is the first metatarsophalangeal joint (podagra), followed by knee, ankle/metatarsus, wrist, and fingers. Polyarticular gout is less common but can occur, in particular in individuals with repeated disease flares. The differential diagnosis of acute gout is wide (**Table 12.1**). It is thus helpful to confirm the diagnosis by demonstrating uric acid crystals in a joint aspirate, ideally during the first episode.

Acute gout is self-limited and symptoms typically resolve over the course of days to weeks. The therapeutic goal during an attack is patient comfort and resolution of inflammation. Several treatment strategies are available (**Table 12.2**). Treatment of the underlying hyperuricemia should not be started during an arthritis flare, because it can prolong the attack.

Table 12.1   Differential Diagnosis of Acute Monoarthritis

Gout
Pseudogout
Septic arthritis and osteomyelitis
Rheumatoid arthritis
Lyme arthritis
Reactive arthritis or other spondyloarthritis
Sarcoidosis
Trauma
Hemarthrosis (e.g., in clotting disorders)
Tumor (pigmented villonodular synovitis, chondrosarcoma)

Table 12.2   Treatment Strategies for Acute Gout

Joint immobilization, with or without analgesics
Nonsteroidal anti-inflammatory drugs
Systemic corticosteroids
Corticosteroid joint injection
Colchicine
IL-1 blocking reagents (experimental)

Intercritical Gout

Most patients with gout are asymptomatic in between sporadic episodes of acute arthritis. The management of patients with intercritical gout focuses on the prevention of further attacks. Interventions include a discussion of lifestyle modifications (avoidance of purine-rich foods, alcohol moderation) and substitution of medications that interfere with uric acid excretion (e.g., diuretics). Other aspects of the metabolic syndrome, when present, should be addressed. Patients should have a "rescue medication" at hand to take when an acute attack begins. Timely intake of a nonsteroidal anti-inflammatory drug (NSAID) at the earliest sign of joint inflammation can significantly reduce the severity and duration of an attack. Chronic NSAIDs or low-dose colchicine reduce the risk for acute gout attacks.

The central question in a patient with intercritical gout is whether to treat the hyperuricemia. Absolute indications for the initiation of uric acid-lowering therapy are provided in **Table 12.3**. Normalization of serum uric acid levels and depletion of body uric acid stores essentially prevent any future gout attack. This needs to be balanced against the requirement for taking a medication for life and the associated risks of drug toxicity.

Table 12.3   Absolute Indications for Uric Acid-Lowering Therapy

Frequent and disabling gout attacks
Polyarticular gout
Tophaceous gout
Kidney stones

Chronic Tophaceous Gout

Untreated gout can lead to severe joint destruction and long-term disability. Tophi are accumulations of uric acid. They can occur in and around joints (often eroding into bone and giving rise to typical "punched-out" lesions on radiograph). Tophi can also be found in the pinna, fingertips, and over the extensor surface of the elbows. Tophaceous gout is an absolute indication for uric acid-lowering therapy.

Workup of the Patient with Acute Gout

In many cases (e.g., classical recurrent podagra in a middle-aged male), the diagnosis of gout poses no diagnostic difficulty, and the workup focuses on determining comorbidities that affect treatment choices. In less clear-cut situations, it is important to rule out alternative diagnoses, in particular a septic joint.

History

A history of acute monoarthritis in a typical joint, previous similar episodes, positive family history, male gender, and older age are suggestive of gout. The presence of precipitating factors such as a high-purine diet or significant alcohol intake should be explored. Postsurgical and hospitalized patients, individuals on diuretic therapy, or those receiving treatment for lymphoproliferative disorders are all at risk.

Atypical joint patterns, prolonged symptom duration, trauma, fever, or chills suggest an alternative diagnosis.

The presence of comorbidities such as renal disease, diabetes mellitus, bleeding disorders, and gastrointestinal bleeding should be investigated, as they affect treatment.

Physical Examination

A complete joint exam should be performed with special attention to the wrists, knees, ankles, and feet. A search should be done for tophi in the pinna, finger joints, fingertips, olecranon bursa, and Achilles tendon. Draining tophaceous material is white and chalky and may look like pus.

Joint Aspiration

A joint aspiration should be attempted during the initial presentation and whenever there is suspicion for a septic joint. Synovial fluid should be sent to the laboratory for gram stain, cell culture, cell count with differential, and crystal exam.

Joint effusions in acute gout are inflammatory (>2000 cells/μl, mostly polymorphonuclear cells). Monosodium uric acid crystals are needle shaped and negatively birefringent under polarized light; intracellular crystals are classical but are not required for the diagnosis (see Figure 12.2).

Laboratory Evaluation

The serum uric acid level can be normal during an acute attack. The erythrocyte sedimentation rate (ESR) and C-reactive protein (CRP) are typically elevated; a mild elevation of the white blood cell count can occur. Complete blood count (CBC), blood urea nitrogen (BUN), creatinine, triglycerides, and glucose are important screens for comorbidities.

Imaging

Radiographs may only show soft tissue swelling. Tophi appear as "punched-out" lesions with overhanging edges. Chronic tophaceous gout may lead to severe joint destruction. Dual-energy computed tomography (CT) can identify uric acid accumulations,[2] but it is not routinely available or done. Ultrasound may detect uric acid deposition on articular surfaces, tophaceous material, and erosions.[3] Imaging cannot reliably distinguish between gout and septic arthritis; joint aspiration must be performed if there is any clinical suspicion.

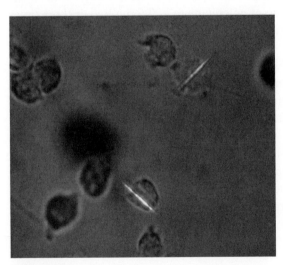

Figure 12.2[9]

Needle-shaped intracellular negatively birefringent crystals consistent with monosodium urate, 400x.

Reproduced from Pascual E and Jovaní V. Synovial fluid analysis. Best Pract Res Clin Rheumatol. 2005;19:371-86.

Management of Acute Gout

An acute gout attack is self-limited. The treatment goal is to accelerate the resolution of symptoms. Several strategies are available, and the treatment selection depends to a large degree on patient comorbidities. NSAIDs and oral corticosteroids are first-choice agents. With few exceptions, treatment strategies for acute gout have not been vigorously tested head-to-head. In one study, 120 patients with acute monoarticular gout were randomized to receive either prednisolone 35 mg daily or naproxen 500 mg twice a day for 5 days. There was no difference in the primary endpoint of pain reduction (measured using a visual analog scale) between both treatment arms.[4]

NSAIDs

A full-dose NSAID (e.g., indomethacin 50 mg three times a day or naproxen 500 mg twice a day) should be scheduled until symptoms resolve. However, contraindications (renal insufficiency, gastrointestinal bleeding, coronary artery disease, hypertension) must be considered.

Systemic Corticosteroids

Oral corticosteroids should be provided at an intermediate dose (e.g., 20 to 40 mg prednisone) and tapered over 1 to 2 weeks. Contraindications should be considered (e.g., brittle diabetes, congestive heart failure, infection).

Corticosteroid Joint Injection

The intra-articular application of an injectable corticosteroid (e.g., methylprednisolone acetate, triamcinolone hexacetonide) circumvents most problems of systemic corticosteroids but carries its own risks (i.e., bleeding, infection). Joint injection requires expertise, and some joints are difficult to inject (including the commonly affected first metatarsophalangeal joint). Consider ultrasound guidance, if available.

Colchicine

The "classical" regimen of 0.6 mg colchicine every hour will cause gastrointestinal upset and diarrhea in most patients.[5] A low dose of colchicine (e.g. 0.6 mg two or three times a day) may be beneficial and more tolerable.

Joint Immobilization

Joint immobilization, with or without analgesics, can be used as adjunct to anti-inflammatory therapies. It can be used as a primary intervention in multimorbid patients with contraindications for the anti-inflammatory agents discussed earlier.

IL-1 Blocking Agents (Experimental)

The use of the recombinant IL-1 receptor antagonist Anakinra was effective for the treatment of acute gout in a small series of patients.[6] Longer-acting IL-1 blockers—Rilonacept (IL-1TRAP) and Canakinumab (a monoclonal anti-IL-1 antibody)—are in clinical trials.

Uric Acid-Lowering Therapies

The indications for initiating uric acid-lowering therapy were discussed earlier (Table 12.3). The most common uric acid-lowering therapies are listed in **Table 12.4.**

Table 12.4   Uric Acid-Lowering Therapies

Xanthine oxidase inhibitors:
- Allopurinol
- Febuxostat

Uricosurica:
- Probenecid

Recombinant uricase:
- Rasburicase
- Pegloticase (PEGylated uricase, FDA approval pending)

Xanthine Oxidase Inhibitors

Allopurinol (Zyloprim) is the most commonly used drug for reducing uric acid levels. Allopurinol inhibits xanthine oxidase, thus reducing uric acid formation. Allopurinol is started in the asymptomatic gout patient. It is common practice to supply the patient with an NSAID or low-dose colchicine in order to prevent induction of an acute gout flare.

The standard dose of allopurinol is 300 mg daily. However, some patients may require considerably higher doses in order to achieve the target serum uric acid concentration of <6 mg/dL. Renal insufficiency is not a contraindication for allopurinol; however, these patients should be started on a lower dose (100 mg daily or less). The allopurinol dose should be titrated until the serum target level is achieved. After a dose change, allow the uric acid level to stabilize over 1 month before repeat testing. Common side effects include nausea/vomiting, skin rash, and leucopenia. Allopurinol hypersensitivity syndrome, which is characterized by dermatitis, hepatitis, and renal failure, is rare.

Febuxostat is a novel nonnucleoside xanthine oxidase inhibitor. It effectively lowers uric acid levels and was recently approved by the FDA. In one study, 1072 subjects with uric acid levels ≥8 mg/dL and serum creatine ≤2 mg/dL were randomized to receive a placebo, Febuxostat (80, 120, or 240 mg daily), or allopurinol (100 or 300 mg daily based on renal function) for 28 weeks. Febuxostat was more effective in achieving a uric acid level of <6 mg/dL than the fixed dose of allopurinol.[7]

Febuxostat is considerably more expensive than allopurinol, but it offers an alternative for patients who cannot tolerate allopurinol. The starting dose is 40 mg daily. The dose is increased to 80 mg daily if the serum uric acid level is still elevated after 2 weeks. Side effects include liver function test abnormalities, nausea, rash, and arthralgias.

Uricosuric Agents

An alternative treatment strategy is the use of drugs that increase renal uric acid excretion. Probenecid is the uricosuric agent currently available in the United States. It should only be given to patients with low 24-hour urinary uric acid excretion and is not effective in patients with a reduced glomerular filtration rate. A history of kidney stones is an absolute contraindication, and patients on this drug should maintain a high urine volume.

The angiotensin receptor blocker losartan and the lipid-lowering drug fenofibrate have mild uricosuric effects. This feature may make these reagents a preferred choice when treating comorbidities.

Recombinant Uricases

A subset of patients with severe tophaceous gout cannot tolerate allopurinol or cannot achieve normalization of their uric acid level even at highest doses. For these patients with "treatment failure" gout, administration of a recombinant uricase might be a treatment option in the future. Rasburicase is already being used for gout prophylaxis in hematologic malignancies.

Pegloticase is less immunogenic and effectively lowers serum uric acid levels in patients with treatment failure gout. In one study, 41 patients with treatment failure gout were randomized to receive repeated Pegloticase infusions at 4 dosage levels for 12 to 14 weeks. Serum uric acid levels were persistently lowered to <6 mg/dL in most participants, 88% of patients experienced a gout flare.[8] Pegloticase is expected to be approved by the FDA in the near future.

Table 12.5   Conditions Associated with pseudogout

Hemochromatosis	Hypophosphatemia
Hypothyroidism	Hyperparathyroidism
Hypomagnesemia	

CALCIUM PYROPHOSPHATE DIHYDRATE DISEASE

Calcium pyrophosphate dihydrate (CPPD) disease comprises a spectrum of inflammatory arthropathies caused by joint deposition of calcium pyrophosphate dihydrate. The most common variant is pseudogout, which is characterized by acute joint inflammation similar to uric acid crystal-induced gout. Less common presentations resemble rheumatoid arthritis (pseudo-RA) or severe destructive osteoarthritis (pseudo-OA). Chondrocalcinosis is the radiographic finding of calcium deposits in cartilage. Chondrocalcinosis is often an incidental radiograph finding; it is not a disease in itself.

Pseudogout presents like gout with an acute monoarthritis. Upper extremity involvement of the wrist is common; knees and ankles can be affected as well. Age is the main risk factor. A diagnosis of pseudogout ideally requires demonstration of CPPD crystals in synovial fluid plus chondrocalcinosis on plain radiograph. Frequently, only one of two findings is present. CPPD and uric acid crystals may coexist in a single patient.

A number of diseases are associated with CPPD: hemochromatosis, hypothyroidism, hypomagnesemia, hypophosphatemia, and hyperparathyroidism. Screening for these potentially treatable conditions is imperative, particularly in younger patients.

Workup of the Patient with Pseudogout

History

A diagnosis of CPPD disease often includes a history of episodic monoarthritis involving the wrists, knees, and ankles. Older age is a risk factor, but the male bias seen in gout is not observed. Hospitalized and postsurgical patients are at risk for this disorder. The practitioner should inquire about metabolic disorders associated with CPPD disease.

Examination

A complete joint exam should be performed if pseudogout is suspected.

Joint Aspiration

Synovial fluid should be sent to the laboratory for gram stain, cell culture, cell count with differential, and crystal examination. Joint effusions in pseudogout are inflammatory (>2000 cells/μl, mostly polymorphs) and may be hemorrhagic. CPPD crystals are rhomboid and demonstrate positive birefringence under polarized light (**Figure 12.3**).

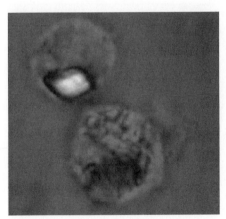

Figure 12.3   Intracellular CPPD crystal[9]

Note the rhomboid shape. CPPD crystals are weakly positively birefringent.

Reproduced from Pascual E & Jovaní V. Synovial fluid analysis. Best Pract Res Clin Rheumatol 2005;19:371-86.

Laboratory

Laboratory findings may demonstrate elevated ESR and CRP levels. Iron, transferrin, ferritin, magnesium, calcium, phosphorus, and thyroid-stimulating hormone should be ordered to screen for metabolic abnormalities associated with CPPD disease.

Imaging

Radiographs of the involved joint may be helpful in ruling out alternative diagnoses. The practitioner should look for chondrocalcinosis on radiographs. This is most often seen in the wrist (triangular cartilage), knee, and symphysis pubis. Ultrasound may reveal cartilage calcifications.

Management

The treatment of acute pseudogout attacks is similar to that of acute gout caused by uric acid crystals. Long-term management consists of treating any underlying metabolic abnormality, when possible. Low-dose colchicine (0.6 mg once or twice daily) may be helpful in preventing disease flares. Chronic arthritis (pseudo-RA) may require treatment with disease-modifying antirheumatic drugs (DMARDs), such as methotrexate.

OTHER CRYSTAL-INDUCED ARTHROPATHIES

Several other types of crystals can be found in the synovial fluid of inflamed joints. These are much less common than uric acid or CPPD crystals.

Basic Calcium Phosphate Crystals

Basic calcium phosphate crystals are too small to be seen with regular light microscopy. They can be demonstrated by electron microscopy, and aggregates stain positive with calcium dyes such as Alizarin Red. However, these tests are not usually performed in clinical practice.

Basic calcium phosphate crystals can be found in a variety of arthropathies, including RA and OA. They tend to occur with more destructive disease. An example for this is the Milwaukee shoulder, a rapidly progressive and highly destructive monoarthropathy that mainly affects elderly women. Basic calcium phosphate crystals can be found in intra- and periarticular distribution.

Oxalate Crystals

Oxalate crystals are very rare. Oxalate crystals can occur as the result of a primary metabolic defect or in patients on hemodialysis.

Cholesterol Crystals

Cholesterol crystals are large and brightly birefringent (**Figure 12.4**). Cholesterol crystals can be present in chronic joint effusions of various etiologies; their presence is of uncertain significance.[9]

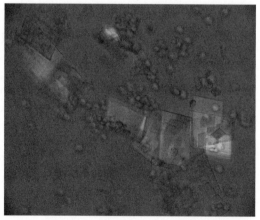

Figure 12.4   Cholesterol crystals

Cholesterol crystals are very large, sheet-like, and birefringent.

Picture courtesy of Dr. Michael Weinblatt.

SUMMARY

Crystal-induced arthropathies are an important consideration in the differential diagnosis of acute monoarticular arthritis. In older and hospitalized patients, the first presentation of both gout and pseudogout can be polyarticular. Joint aspiration, with fluid sent for cell count, gram stain, and culture to rule out infection, should be performed whenever possible to confirm a diagnosis of crystal-induced arthropathy. Acute management of gout and pseudogout includes NSAIDs, colchicine, and corticosteroids. Other experimental therapies are being explored. Long-term management of gouty arthritis focuses on lowering the serum uric acid level, whereas long-term management of pseudogout targets comorbidities and may in some cases involve more traditional DMARDs.

◇◇◇◇◇◇◇◇◇◇◇◇

REFERENCES

1. Feig DI, Kang DH, Johnson RJ. Uric acid and cardio-vascular risk. *N Engl J Med.* 2008;359:1811–1121.
2. Choi HK, Al-Arfaj A, Eftekhari A, et al. Dual-energy computed tomography in tophaceous gout. *Ann Rheum Dis.* 2009;68:1609–1612.
3. Thiele RG, Schlesinger N. Diagnosis of gout by ultrasound. *Rheumatology (Oxford).* 2007;46:1116–1121.
4. Janssens HJ, Janssen M, van de Lisdonk EH, van Riel PL, van Weel C. Use of oral prednisolone or naproxen for the treatment of gout arthritis: a double-blind, randomised equivalence trial. *Lancet.* 2008;371:1854–1860.
5. Ahern MJ, Reid C, Gordon TP, McCredie M, Brooks PM, Jones M. Does colchicine work? The results of the first controlled study in acute gout. *Aust N Z J Med.* 1987;17:301–304.
6. So A, De Smedt T, Revaz S, Tschopp J. A pilot study of IL-1 inhibition by anakinra in acute gout. *Arthritis Res Ther.* 2007;9:R28.
7. Schumacher HR, Becker MA, Wortmann RL, et al. Effects of febuxostat versus allopurinol and placebo in reducing serum urate in subjects with hyperuricemia and gout: a 28-week, phase III, randomized, double-blind, parallel-group trial. *Arthritis Rheum.* 2008;59:1540–1548.
8. Sundy JS, Becker MA, Baraf HS, et al. Reduction of plasma urate levels following treatment with multiple doses of pegloticase (polyethylene glycol-conjugated uricase) in patients with treatment-failure gout: Results of a phase II randomized study. *Arthritis Rheum.* 2008;58:2882–2891.
9. Pascual E, Jovaní V. Synovial fluid analysis. *Best Pract Res Clin Rheumatol.* 2005;19:371–386.

CHAPTER 13

Infectious Arthritis

Katherine P. Liao, MD

OVERVIEW

Infectious arthritis should be suspected in any adult presenting with acute mono- or oligoarticular arthritis. Patients may also present with polyarticular septic arthritis, especially elderly patients and/or those who are immunocompromised. The three major groups of infectious arthritides are: bacterial (nongonococcal), bacterial (gonococcal), and Lyme arthritis. A summary of the organisms and populations at risk are summarized in **Table 13.1**.

Table 13.1   Causes of Infectious Arthritis in Adults

	PATHOGEN	POPULATION
Bacterial (nongonococcal)		
Gram positive	*Staphylococcus aureus*	Most common in all populations
	Streptococcus: pneumonia, group A *streptococcus*	Second most common in healthy individuals
	Staphylococcus epidermidis	Post-instrumentation
Gram-negative rods	*Pseudomonas aeruginosa*	Intravenous drug users Immunocompromised patients Persons with prosthetic joints
	Salmonella	Persons with sickle cell disease
Bacterial (gonococcal)		
Gram-negative cocci	*Neisseria gonorrhea*	Young, sexually active adults Male: female (1:3)
Lyme		
Spirochete	*Borrelia burgdorferi*	Healthy individuals living in endemic areas of the U.S.: northeast from Maine to Maryland; midwest in Wisconsin and Minnesota; west in northern California and Oregon

(continues)

Table 13.1   Causes of Infectious Arthritis in Adults, cont'd

	PATHOGEN	POPULATION
Other		
	Mycobacteria and fungi	Immunocompromised patients
	Viral	Healthy individuals

This chapter will discuss the major pathogens involved in infectious arthritis, discuss at-risk populations, and review the clinical features, diagnosis, and treatment of these conditions.

BACTERIAL (NONGONOCOCCAL) ARTHRITIS

Infection of the joint can theoretically be caused by any organism and can occur through three routes: (1) direct inoculation (i.e., via bite, trauma, or instrumentation); (2) contiguous spread from infected bone or soft tissue; or (3) through hematogenous spread. Joint infections are typically caused by one organism. Polymicrobial joint infections, when they occur, are usually the result of open wounds or trauma.

The organism most often involved in joint infections in adults is *Staphylococcus aureus* (*S. aureus*). Streptococci, including *S. pneumonia* and group A *streptococcus*, are the second most common pathogens. Gram-negative infections, such as those from *Pseudomonas* and *E. coli* are less common. These pathogens are most commonly found in intravenous drug users, the elderly, diabetics, and those with major immune deficiencies.[1] In sickle cell patients, *Salmonella* infection should also be considered.

Risk Factors

General risk factors for joint infection include previously damaged joints, infection at another site in the body, and chronic illnesses that predispose to infection, such as malignancies, diabetes, cirrhosis, and HIV. Intravenous drug users (IVDU) are also at high risk due to seeding of joints from bacteremia.

A review of patients who presented with acute painful swollen joints found specific risk factors that substantially increased the relative risk (RR) of bacterial arthritis as the cause:[2]

- Recent joint surgery (RR 8.4)
- Rheumatoid arthritis (RR 5.4)
- Age >80 years (RR 4.1)
- Hip or knee prosthesis (RR 4.1)

- Skin infection (RR 3.6)
- HIV (RR 3.2)
- Diabetes mellitus (RR 2.8)

Laboratory Studies

Arthrocentesis is the definitive diagnostic test for all suspected cases of bacterial arthritis. An 18- or 16-gauge needle should be used to allow for aspiration of purulent material. Hip or shoulder joints commonly require aspiration under fluoroscopy or ultrasound guidance. The synovial fluid should analyzed for gram stain (priority, with culture, if insufficient fluid for all tests), culture, cell count with differential, and crystals. All synovial fluid should also be examined for the presence of crystals. The presence of crystals does not rule out an infection, because both processes can coexist in the same joint. Immunocompromised patients require the following, additional tests: fungal stain and culture and acid fast bacilli (AFB) stain and cultures.

Peripheral blood cultures and complete cell count should also be obtained; blood cultures can be positive in up to 50% of cases of septic arthritis. Other cultures, such as sputum and urine, should be obtained if infection is also suspected at these sites.

Imaging

Radiographs of the affected joint should be obtained. Destructive changes are not usually present early in the disease course (days to weeks). However, if destructive changes consistent with infectious arthritis or osteomyelitis are present, aggressive intervention (surgical intervention) and prolonged antibiotic coverage may be warranted. For joints that are difficult to visualize—for example, the hip—computed tomography (CT) or magnetic resonance imaging (MRI) is recommended to assess for inflammation and the presence of an effusion.

Diagnosis

Identification of a causative organism from joint cultures provides a definitive diagnosis of septic arthritis. However, if clinical suspicion is high, a patient should be treated for a septic joint even in the absence of positive cultures.

Synovial fluid white blood cell (WBC) counts >50,000/mm³ are highly suspicious for infection in immunocompetent patients. Septic joints can have lower WBC counts (<5000/mm³); in particular, patients with gonococcal arthritis and tuberculous arthritis may have low joint fluid WBC counts. In most cases, the joint fluid has >90% polymorphonuclear cells (PMNs). Synovial fluid glucose and protein levels are nonspecific for septic arthritis and are no longer recommended as routine tests in the initial evaluation of a septic joint.[3]

Treatment

If a bacterial arthritis is suspected, treatment should begin ideally after cultures are obtained from the blood and synovial fluid. Initial treatment is empiric and depends upon the patient's risk factors. Therapy should be targeted once information is available from gram stain and cultures. A treatment guide is outlined in **Table 13.2.** In general, all empiric coverage should include antibiotics effective against *S. aureus*.

Empiric coverage for healthy individuals from communities where methicillin-resistant *S. aureus* (MRSA) is not a concern includes bactericidal agents such as nafcillin or oxacillin. If MRSA is a concern, coverage should include vancomycin and a third-generation cephalosporin. Similarly, if there is concern for gram-negative infection, such as in IVDU, diabetics, or immunocompromised patients, vancomycin and a third-generation cephalosporin are recommended.

Duration of treatment ranges from 2 to 6 weeks (or longer) and is dependent on the pathogen, clinical response to therapy, and underlying joint damage.

There are no prospective data comparing serial closed needle aspiration, arthroscopic drainage, and arthrotomy. Surgical intervention is generally preferred in the following situations:

- Infection in weight-bearing joints (i.e., hip)
- Joint not accessible to percutaneous aspiration (i.e., hip, shoulder)
- Loculated fluid in joint space
- Imaging studies show evidence of joint damage

Infected prosthetic implants almost always require removal to eradicate infection, in addition to targeted antibiotic treatment. In rare instances (frail host) and with certain bacteria (group A *streptococcus*), prolonged antibiotic suppression may be administered without removal of the prosthesis. Additional coverage with rifampin is often used for its bactericidal activity against biofilm-producing bacteria in combination with a fluoroquinolone.[4]

Table 13.2   Antibiotic Regimens for Bacterial Arthritis According to Suspected Organism[5]

Pathogen	Treatment	Comment
S. aureus	Nafcillin or oxacillin (2 g, IV, every 4 hours)	No MRSA risk factors
S. aureus (MRSA risk)	Vancomycin (1 g, IV, every 12 hours)	

(continues)

Table 13.2 Antibiotic Regimens for Bacterial Arthritis According to Suspected Organism,[5] cont'd

PATHOGEN	TREATMENT	COMMENT
P. aeruginosa	Ceftazidime or Cefepime (2 g, every 8 hours)	IVDU
N. gonorrhea	Ceftriaxone (1 g, IV, every 12 hours) or Cefotaxime (1 g, IV, every 8 hours)	Treat presumptively for chlamydia (doxycycline, 100 mg daily for 7 days)
Empiric coverage for gram-positive and gram-negative organisms	Vancomycin (1 g, IV, every 12 hours) + Ceftazidime (2 g, IV, every 8 hours) or Cefepime (2 g, IV, every 12 hours) or Piperacillin/tazobactam (4.5 g, IV, every 6 hours)	Health-care associated, MRSA, IVDU

Adapted from Johns Hopkins Antibiotic Guide.

Bacterial arthritis has a mortality of 10 to 15% and carries a high morbidity with irreversible loss of joint function in 25 to 50% of surviving patients.[6]

DISSEMINATED GONOCOCCAL INFECTION

Disseminated gonococcal infection (DGI) caused by *Neisseria gonorrhea* is the most common cause of infectious arthritis in young, sexually active adults. The pathogen is transmitted sexually; women are affected three times more than men. Risk factors for dissemination in women include menstruation, pregnancy, or the postpartum state,[7] and, for both genders, systemic lupus erythematosus and deficiencies in complement.[8]

Patients with DGI tend to present with either of two syndromes:

- Bacteremia with the triad of polyarthritis, tenosynovitis, and skin lesions, without joint effusions
- Purulent arthritis (40%) affecting the knees, wrists, hands, and/or ankles[9]

Patients who have bacteremia present with a prodrome of fever, malaise, and migratory polyarthralgias. These patients often have acute onset of tenosynovitis (>60%) in the wrists, fingers, ankles, and toes. Skin lesions (>60%) appear as gunmetal-gray pustules with an erythematous base on the extremities and trunk.[9] These lesions are transient, typically painless, and persist for 3 to 4 days. Other rare dermatologic manifestations associated with DGI include erythema nodosum and erythema multiforme.[10]

The joint-localized form of the disease, purulent arthritis, typically involves one or two joints, particularly the knees, wrists, or ankles. Most patients are afebrile and lack signs of systemic disease and/or infections at other sites.[10] Less commonly, patients can have a combination of both syndromes.

Laboratory Studies

If a joint effusion is present, arthrocentesis should be used to confirm the diagnosis. As in all cases where bacterial infection is suspected, a gram stain, culture and cell count should be obtained. Patients with clinical features of polyarthritis, tenosynovitis, and skin lesions should also have cultures of the skin lesions, urethra, or cervix. Cultures can also be obtained from the pharynx and rectum if the patient is symptomatic. All cultures should be done on Thayer-Martin media. Blood cultures should also be obtained.

Diagnosis

A patient should be treated for DGI if the history and physical exam are consistent, regardless of culture results, because the sensitivity of gram stain and culture from the synovial fluid for gonococcal arthritis can be low, ranging from 10 to 25% and 10 to 50%, respectively.[11] A positive gram stain or culture is highly specific and would confirm the diagnosis. Synovial fluid WBC counts generally range from 40,000 to 60,000/mm^3 with PMN predominance of >80%.

Treatment[12]

Initial treatment includes one of the following regimen:

- Ceftriaxone (1 g, intramuscular or intravenous, every 24 hours)
- Cefotaxime (1 g, intravenous, every 8 hours)
- Ceftizoxime (1 g, intravenous, every 8 hours)

If there is improvement from the initial therapy after 24 to 48 hours, the patient can be switched to oral therapy to complete 1 week total of antibiotic therapy:

- Cefixime (400 mg, by mouth, twice a day)

OR

- Cefpodoxime (400 mg, by mouth, twice a day)

The patient should also be treated presumptively for chlamydia with 100 mg of doxycycline by mouth for 7 days. When possible, sexual partners of patients with DGI should be treated. Fluoroquinolones are no longer recommended due to increasing resistance.

LYME ARTHRITIS

Lyme disease, caused by *Borrelia burgdorferi*, is the most common tick-borne infection in the United States. It is transmitted by the tick species *Ixodes scapularis* and *Ixodes pacificus*. The infection typically requires tick attachment for 36 to 48 hours before the disease is transmitted to the human host.[13]

The disease is endemic in the northeast from Maine to Maryland, in the midwest in Wisconsin and Minnesota, and in the west in northern California and Oregon and is often contracted in fields and forested areas.[14] Peak incidence of the disease occurs in the summer months between May and August.

Clinical Manifestations

The infection can involve multiple organs and is considered to have three stages with associated signs and symptoms (**Table 13.3**).

Table 13.3   Stages and Clinical Manifestations of Lyme Disease

STAGE	DURATION	CLINICAL MANIFESTATIONS
Stage 1: Early localized disease Local infection by spirochete	Days	Flu-like illness Erythema chronicum migrans (ECM)*
Stage 2: Early disseminated disease Spirochetemia and immune response	Days to weeks	Constitutional symptoms: fever, malaise, headache, and lymphadenopathy Migratory arthralgias, mono- or oligoarthritis Myalgias Facial nerve palsy Carditis/conduction abnormalities
Stage 3: Late persistent	Months to years	Recurrent mono or oligoarthritis of large joints Acrodermatitis chronica atropicans Polyneuropathy

*ECM is a macular erythematous lesion with central clearing; mean size of lesion 15 cm (range 3 to 78 cm).

Lyme arthritis is typically mono- or oligoarticular and most commonly affects the knee, shoulder, and ankle. After the appearance of erythema chronicum migrans (ECM) in untreated individuals, 80% of individuals will develop migratory arthralgias approximately 2 weeks after the onset of the rash (1 day to 8 weeks).[15,16] Patients with persistent disease can develop mono- or oligoarticular arthritis with effusions.

Diagnosis

The diagnosis of early Lyme disease can be made clinically from the presence of ECM in a patient who lives in an endemic area. It does not require laboratory confirmation.[17]

Serum

If a patient has clinical signs or symptoms that are consistent with Lyme disease (pretest probability >20%), a serologic test has high clinical utility. Serologic testing in individuals with nonspecific symptoms who do not live or have not traveled in endemic areas (pretest probability <20%) can lead to misleading results due to the high rate of false-positive tests.

CDC guidelines recommend a two-tier testing system for Lyme. If the enzyme-linked immunosorbent assay screening (ELISA) (sensitivity 89%, specificity 72%) is positive, a confirmative Western Blot (IgM and IgG immunoblots) is conducted. If the ELISA screening is negative, no further testing is required. False-positive results can be due to other spirochetal diseases; autoimmune diseases, such as SLE; and viral illnesses, such as Epstein-Barr and HIV. The screening ELISA can be negative in early Lyme disease if testing occurs before the production of antibodies. However, a negative-screening ELISA virtually rules out the presence of the disease in patients who are concerned about persistent disease, because positive titers are present several years after the initial infection (after 20 years, 62% had positive IgG titers to Lyme in some studies).[18,19]

In addition, blood cultures, a complete blood count (CBC), and liver function tests should be performed to rule out other possible infectious causes. All patients should be evaluated for coinfection with *Babesia* and *Ehrlichia*.

Synovial Fluid

Arthrocentesis is recommended to rule out other infectious or inflammatory causes. Synovial white blood cell (WBC) counts in Lyme disease average from 21,000 to 24,000 cell/mm^3 with a PMN predominance.[15]

Polymerase chain reaction (PCR) of the synovial fluid is an option, however, the clinical test results can be variable and false-positives are common.[20] The test is most useful in the setting of arthritis symptoms in those with seropositive results with minimal or no response to treatment. A positive result does not necessarily confirm active disease, as the amplified DNA can be obtained from live organisms or remnants of a prior infection.[21] The yield is higher in untreated patients (97%) than in treated patients (37%).[22]

Differential Diagnosis

Recently, a Lyme-like illness, southern tick-associated rash illness (STARI), has been characterized. The causative organism from this illness has not been identified, but the vector has been identified as the Lone Star tick (*Amblyomma americanum*).[23] Arthritis symptoms have been reported to be less severe than Lyme.

Treatment

The Infectious Diseases Society of America (IDSA) guidelines for the treatment of Lyme disease are detailed in **Tables 13.4** and **13.5**. Lyme arthritis (clear evidence of joint swelling) can be treated with an oral regimen of doxycycline, amoxicillin, or cefuroxime. Approximately 90% of patients with Lyme arthritis will respond to a single course of oral therapy.[24]

Table 13.4   Recommended Antimicrobial Treatment for Lyme Disease[13]

MEDICATION	DOSE
Oral	
Doxycycline	100 mg twice a day
Cefuroxime	500 mg twice a day
Amoxicillin	500 mg three times a day
Parenteral	
Ceftriaxone	2 g, IV, four times a day

Adapted from Wormser, et al.

Table 13.5   Treatment According to Stage of Disease and Clinical Manifestation

STAGE OF DISEASE	TREATMENT	DURATION DAYS (RANGE)
Tick bite in endemic area	Doxycycline (200 mg, by mouth)	One
Early		
ECM	Oral	14 (14–21)
Early disseminated		
Neurologic: meningitis, cranial nerve palsy	Parenteral/oral	14 (10–28)/14 (14–21)
Cardiac disease	Oral/parenteral	14 (14–21)
Late		
Arthritis without neurologic symptoms	Oral	28

(continues)

Table 13.5   Treatment According to Stage of Disease and Clinical Manifestation, cont'd

STAGE OF DISEASE	TREATMENT	DURATION DAYS (RANGE)
Recurrent arthritis after oral regimen	Oral/parenteral	28/14 (14–28)
Antibiotic refractory arthritis	Symptomatic therapy; consider hydroxychloroquine	
Central or peripheral nervous system	Parenteral	14 (14–28)
Acrodermatitis chronic atrophicans	Oral	21 (14–28)

Although oral therapy is generally well tolerated, 12% of patients can experience transient worsening of symptoms 24 hours after treatment, attributed to the Jarisch-Herxheimer reaction.[25,26]

In rare cases, patients with documented Lyme arthritis who no longer have evidence of persistent infection can experience persistent synovitis despite appropriate oral and/or intravenous antibiotic therapy. Treatment with mild-to-moderate immunosuppressive medications such as hydroxycholoroquine or methotrexate has been effective in this group. For patients who continue to have synovitis despite 3 to 6 months of immunosuppressive therapy, surgical management with synovectomy is also an option.[15]

OTHER CAUSES OF INFECTIOUS ARTHRITIS

Mycobacterial and Fungal Arthritis

In immunocompromised patients, joint infection with mycobacteria and fungal arthritis must be considered. The onset is generally insidious, with a predilection for the spine and weight-bearing joints. Although swelling is usually present, signs of acute joint inflammation such as erythema and warmth are not.

Laboratory Studies

If a joint effusion is present, arthrocentesis should be done and fluid sent for AFB smear/culture and fungal stain/culture in addition to gram stain/culture to confirm the diagnosis. A synovial tissue biopsy should also be considered, especially when there is a small amount of synovial fluid.

Diagnosis

Synovial fluid WBC counts generally range between 10,000 to 30,000 cell/mm^3 in both fungal and mycobacterial arthritis. A wide range in the percentage of positive cultures appears in the literature. Synovial tissue cultures appear to be the most reliable for these insidious infections and are positive in >90% for both pathogens.[1]

Treatment

Mycobacterial antibiotics and antifungal agents used to treat systemic disease are generally effective in eradicating joint infection. However, surgical joint debridement may be necessary.[1]

Viral Arthritis

Viral arthritides typically present with polyarthritis in adults, in contrast to monoarthritis seen in bacterial infections. Patients can present with symmetric arthritis involving the hand, a physical finding atypical of septic arthritis. The most common causative agent is Parvovirus B19.

Parvovirus B19 infections peak in late winter and early spring. This infection commonly occurs in individuals who have exposure to young children. Rheumatologic manifestations in the adult include a lacy reticular rash on the lower extremities and an inflammatory arthritis that is indistinguishable from rheumatoid arthritis. Symptoms usually resolve after 6 months. Other causes of viral arthritis include rubella (following infection or immunization)[27] and mumps (predominantly in adult males). Arthritis can also develop in individuals infected with hepatitis B prior to development of jaundice and in hepatitis C with cryoglobulinemia. HIV can present with arthralgias of multiple joints and rarely, monoarthritis.[28]

◇◇◇◇◇◇◇◇◇◇◇◇

REFERENCES

1. Goldenberg DL. Septic arthritis. *Lancet.* 1998;351(9097):197–202.
2. Margaretten ME, Kohlwes J, Moore D, Bent S. Does this adult patient have septic arthritis? *JAMA.* 2007;297(13):1478–1488.
3. Shmerling RH, Delbanco TL, Tosteson AN, Trentham DE. Synovial fluid tests. What should be ordered? *JAMA.* 1990;264(8):1009–1014.
4. Zimmerli W, Trampuz A, Ochsner PE. Prosthetic-joint infections. *N Engl J Med.* 2004;351(16):1645–1654.
5. Bartlett JG (ed). *Johns Hopkins Antibiotic Guide.* http://prod.hopkins-abxguide.org; 2007.
6. Kaandorp CJ, Krijnen P, Moens HJ, Habbema JD, van Schaardenburg D. The outcome of bacterial arthritis: a prospective community-based study. *Arthritis Rheum.* 1997;40(5):884–892.
7. Phupong V, Sittisomwong T, Wisawasukmongchol W. Disseminated gonococcal infection during pregnancy. *Arch Gynecol Obstet.* 2005;273(3):185–186.
8. Petersen BH, Lee TJ, Snyderman R, Brooks GF. Neisseria meningitidis and Neisseria gonorrhoeae bacteremia associated with C6, C7, or C8 deficiency. *Ann Intern Med.* 1979;90(6):917–920.

9. O'Brien JP, Goldenberg DL, Rice PA. Disseminated gonococcal infection: a prospective analysis of 49 patients and a review of pathophysiology and immune mechanisms. *Medicine (Baltimore)*. 1983;62(6):395–406.

10. Rice PA. Gonococcal arthritis (disseminated gonococcal infection). *Infect Dis Clin North Am.* 2005;19(4):853–861.

11. Brannan SR, Jerrard DA. Synovial fluid analysis. *J Emerg Med.* 2006;30(3):331–339.

12. Centers for Disease Control and Prevention, Updated recommended treatment regimens for gonococcal infections and associated conditions—United States; April 2007. http://www.cdc.gov/STD/treatment/.

13. Wormser GP, Dattwyler RJ, Shapiro ED, et al. The clinical assessment, treatment, and prevention of Lyme disease, human granulocytic anaplasmosis, and babesiosis: clinical practice guidelines by the Infectious Diseases Society of America. *Clin Infect Dis.* 2006;43(9):1089–1134.

14. Steere AC. Lyme disease. *N Engl J Med.* 2001;345(2):115–125.

15. Puius YA, Kalish RA. Lyme arthritis: pathogenesis, clinical presentation, and management. *Infect Dis Clin North Am.* 2008;22(2):289–300, vi–vii.

16. Steere AC, Schoen RT, Taylor E. The clinical evolution of Lyme arthritis. *Ann Intern Med.* 1987;107(5):725–731.

17. Guidelines for laboratory evaluation in the diagnosis of Lyme disease. American College of Physicians. *Ann Intern Med.* 1997;127(12):1106–1108.

18. Feder HM Jr., Gerber MA, Luger SW, Ryan RW. Persistence of serum antibodies to *Borrelia burgdorferi* in patients treated for Lyme disease. *Clin Infect Dis.* 1992;15(5):788–793.

19. Kalish RA, Kaplan RF, Taylor E, Jones-Woodward L, Workman K, Steere AC. Evaluation of study patients with Lyme disease, 10–20-year follow-up. *J Infect Dis.* 2001;183(3):453–60.

20. Nocton JJ, Dressler F, Rutledge BJ, Rys PN, Persing DH, Steere AC. Detection of *Borrelia burgdorferi* DNA by polymerase chain reaction in synovial fluid from patients with Lyme arthritis. *N Engl J Med.* 1994;330(4):229–234.

21. Sigal LH. The polymerase chain reaction assay for *Borrelia burgdorferi* in the diagnosis of Lyme disease. *Ann Intern Med.* 1994;120(6):520–521.

22. Aguero-Rosenfeld ME. Lyme disease: laboratory issues. *Infect Dis Clin North Am.* 2008;22(2):301–313, vii.

23. Masters EJ, Grigery CN, Masters RW. STARI, or Masters disease: Lone Star tick-vectored Lyme-like illness. *Infect Dis Clin North Am.* 2008;22(2):361–376, viii.

24. Steere AC, Levin RE, Molloy PJ, et al. Treatment of Lyme arthritis. *Arthritis Rheum.* 1994;37(6):878–888.

25. Luger SW, Paparone P, Wormser GP, et al. Comparison of cefuroxime axetil and doxycycline in treatment of patients with early Lyme disease associated with erythema migrans. *Antimicrob Agents Chemother.* 1995;39(3):661–667.

26. Massarotti EM, Luger SW, Rahn DW, et al. Treatment of early Lyme disease. *Am J Med.* 1992;92(4):396–403.

27. Calabrese LH, Naides SJ. Viral arthritis. *Infect Dis Clin North Am.* 2005;19(4):963–980, x.

28. Smith JW, Chalupa P, Shabaz Hasan M. Infectious arthritis: clinical features, laboratory findings and treatment. *Clin Microbiol Infect.* 2006;12(4):309–314.

CHAPTER 14
Miscellaneous Rheumatic Diseases

Rumey Ishizawar, MD

OVERVIEW

This chapter presents overviews of four rheumatic diseases: scleroderma, idiopathic inflammatory myositis, Sjogren's syndrome, and relapsing polychondritis. The discussion focuses on the diagnosis, clinical manifestations, pathogenesis, and available treatments for each of these conditions.

SCLERODERMA

Scleroderma (systemic sclerosis) is an autoimmune-mediated heterogeneous disorder characterized by fibrosis of the skin and internal organs with resultant vascular damage. The two main subgroups of scleroderma are limited cutaneous scleroderma and diffuse cutaneous scleroderma. Scleroderma is a rare disorder with an estimated incidence of 2.3 to 22.8 cases per 1 million persons per year and a prevalence of 50 to 300 cases per 1 million persons. Systemic sclerosis commonly affects females more than males, with the estimated ratio ranging between 3:1 and 14:1. Mean age at diagnosis is between the third and fourth decade of life.

Diagnosis

Due to the heterogeneity of scleroderma, diagnosis may be difficult. The differential diagnosis of diseases with clinical manifestations of skin fibrosis or thickening is noted in **Table 14.1**. The American College of Rheumatology (ACR) devised a criteria scheme for scleroderma classification in 1980 that has been externally validated (**Table 14.2**). In the original study, the ACR classification criteria was noted to be 97% sensitive and 98% specific, but subsequent utilization of the criteria in different patient registries found that it had an approximate sensitivity of 70% for diagnosis.

In recent years, the ACR scleroderma classification criteria have also been challenged due to the development of other diagnostic methods, such as identification of autoantibodies, which were not included in the original classification. Although many scleroderma classification criteria have been proposed since 1980, no one set of criteria has been universally accepted. In addition to skin changes, criteria proposed in recent years incorporate autoantibodies, such as anti-CENP, anti-Scl70, anti-RNAP I, anti-RNAP III, anti-fibrillarin, and anti-fibrillin I, as well as microvascular changes noted by nailfold capillaroscopy.

Table 14.1   Differential Diagnosis of Sclerosing Skin Diseases[1]

Systemic sclerosis
- Limited
- Diffuse

Scleromyxedema

Scleredema

Endocrine-associated
- Diabetic cheiroarthropathy
- Hypothyroidism myxedema

Eosinophilic fasciitis

Nephrogenic systemic fibrosis

Amyloidosis

Chemical-induced
- Polyvinyl chloride
- Organic solvents

Drug-induced
- Bleomycin
- D-Penicillamine

Graft-vs-host disease

Adapted from Foti et al., 2008.

Table 14.2   ACR Preliminary Classification Criteria for Scleroderma[2]*

1. Major criteria
   a. Proximal scleroderma

2. Minor criteria
   a. Sclerodactyly
   b. Digital pitting scars or loss of substance at fingertips
   c. Bibasilar pulmonary fibrosis

*Criteria achieved if major criteria or two or more of minor criteria present.

Adapted from Masi et al., 1980.

Clinical Manifestations

Systemic sclerosis typically manifests with skin thickening. In limited cutaneous scleroderma, skin thickening occurs distally, limited to the hands, face, and neck, and patients rarely progress to involve visceral organs. Additional manifestations of limited cutaneous scleroderma include skin calcifications, Raynaud's phenomena, esophageal dysmotility, sclerodactyly, and telangectasia (CREST). In diffuse cutaneous scleroderma, skin thickening occurs more widely and involves more proximal regions of the body. Patients with diffuse cutaneous scleroderma are more likely to have involvement of internal organs and vascular damage. One of the most worrisome clinical manifestations of systemic sclerosis is involvement of the renal vasculature, resulting in scleroderma renal crisis. Scleroderma renal crisis is a medical emergency and early recognition and treatment with an angiotensin-converting enzyme inhibitor can significantly improve life expectancy and decrease the chances for long-term renal replacement therapy. In addition to the kidneys and vasculature, systemic sclerosis can also involve the heart, lung, gastrointestinal tract, as well as the nervous system. With early and aggressive treatment of renal disease, the main morbidity and mortality results from pulmonary and cardiac involvement. The various clinical manifestations of systemic sclerosis are listed in **Table 14.3**.

Table 14.3 Clinical Manifestations of Systemic Sclerosis[3–5]

ORGAN SYSTEM	SIGNS/SYMPTOMS
Skin	Limited/diffuse skin thickening, calcinosis cutis
Gastrointestinal	Dysphagia, esophageal reflux, dysmotility or hypomotility, pseudo-obstruction, bacterial overgrowth, fecal incontinence
Musculoskeletal	Arthralgia, myopathy, osteolysis, avascular necrosis
Vasculature	Raynaud's phenomena, pulmonary artery hypertension, renal crisis
Pulmonary	Interstitial lung disease, aspiration pneumonitis secondary to pharyngeal weakness, bronchoalveolar cell carcinoma
Cardiac	Pericarditis, myocarditis, endocarditis, pulmonary hypertension
Renal	Glomerulonephritis, interstitial nephritis
Neurologic	Neuropathies, autonomic dysfunction

Created with information from Walker et al., 2007, Shah et al., 2008, and Steen VD, 2008.

Pathogenesis

The events that trigger scleroderma in individuals remain unidentified. Hormonal, genetic, and environmental factors are all thought to contribute. Scleroderma is believed to progress in stages, with vascular damage occurring early, followed by mononuclear cell infiltration, and fibrosis occurring later. Cytokines and growth factors are being investigated for their role in endothelial damage, mononuclear cell recruitment, and activation of fibroblasts in remodeling collagen and extracellular matrix leading to fibrosis. Like many autoimmune-related diseases, autoantibodies have been identified in association with scleroderma. The relationship of the autoantibodies to disease mechanism has not been determined; however, they are helpful in diagnosis and predicting disease given specific clinical phenotypes. **Table 14.4** lists the best characterized scleroderma-associated autoantibodies.

Table 14.4   Scleroderma-Specific Autoantibodies[6,7]

AUTOANTIBODIES	CLINICAL PHENOTYPE
Anti-Scl70 (Topoisomerase I)	Diffuse cutaneous scleroderma, interstitial lung disease, cardiac manifestations
Anti-centromere proteins B/C	Limited cutaneous scleroderma, pulmonary hypertension, digital ulcerations, sicca
Anti-RNA polymerase I/II	Diffuse cutaneous scleroderma, renal crisis
Anti-PM/Scl	Polymyositis, sclerosis, calcinosis
Anti-U3RNP (Fibrillarin)	Diffuse cutaneous scleroderma, pulmonary hypertension, cardiac manifestations
Anti-Th/To	Limited cutaneous scleroderma, interstitial lung disease, renal crisis, and gastrointestinal involvement

Adapted from Gabrielli et al., 2009 and Harris et al., 2003.

Treatment

Due to the wide variety of potential manifestations of scleroderma, treatment is directed at symptoms and affected organs. No definitive cure is available for systemic sclerosis, and most treatment is directed at preventing disease progression. Recently, the European League Against Rheumatism (EULAR) Scleroderma Trial and Research (EUSTAR) Group have provided recommendations for the treatment of systemic sclerosis. Recommendations are directed at systemic sclerosis-related digital vasculopathy, pulmonary artery hypertension, skin thickening, interstitial lung disease, renal crisis, and gastrointestinal disease. These recommendations, which are based on evidence-based literature and consensus-driven expert opinions, are listed in **Table 14.5**. In addition to these recommendations, ongoing clinical research testing continues on additional immunosuppressive and cytotoxic therapeutic modalities, as well as other treatments, such as stem cell transplantations.

Summary

Scleroderma (systemic sclerosis) is a heterogeneous autoimmune disorder affecting the vasculature as well as leading to fibrosis of organs. Skin thickening is a key feature of scleroderma, but many other disorders have a similar phenotype. Patients with diffuse

Table 14.5 EULAR/EUSTAR Recommendations for Scleroderma Treatment[8]

1. Digital vasculopathy (Raynaud's phenomenon, digital ulcerations)
   a. Dihidropiridine-type calcium antagonists (oral nifedipine) recommended as first-line therapy for scleroderma-related Raynaud's phenomena.
   b. Intravenous prostanoids (iloprost) recommended for severe Raynaud's phenomenon and treatment of active digital ulcerations.
   c. Bosentan may be considered in diffuse cutaneous scleroderma with multiple digital ulcerations if both calcium antagonists and IV prostanoids have failed.
   d. Phosphodiesterase inhibitors such as sildanafil may be very effective for refractory cases.

2. Pulmonary artery hypertension (PAH)
   a. Bosentan, sitaxentan, and sildanafil have all been shown to improve exercise capacity, functional class, and some hemodynamic measurements in PAH, and may be considered as treatment modality for scleroderma-related PAH.
   b. Continuous intravenous epoprostenol has been shown to improve exercise capacity, functional class, and hemodynamic measurements in PAH, but sudden withdrawal may be life-threatening. Therefore, IV epoprostenol should be considered for severe scleroderma-related PAH.

3. Scleroderma-related skin disease
   a. Methotrexate may be used to treated skin manifestations of early diffuse systemic sclerosis.

4. Interstitial lung disease
   a. Cyclophosphamide is recommended for the treatment of scleroderma-related interstitial lung disease.

5. Scleroderma renal crisis
   a. Angiotensin-converting enzyme (ACE) inhibitors should be utilized in the treatment of scleroderma renal crisis.
   b. Scleroderma patients on steroid therapy should be monitored closely for development of renal crisis by measuring blood pressure and renal function.

6. Gastrointestinal disease
   a. Proton pump inhibitors are recommended to prevent scleroderma-related gastroesophageal reflux disease (GERD) and formation of esophageal ulcers and strictures.
   b. Prokinetic drugs may be helpful for motility disturbances such as dysphagia, early satiety, bloating, and pseudo-obstruction.
   c. Antibiotic therapy with rotational use may be helpful in treating malabsorption from bacterial overgrowth.

Modified from Kowal-Bielecka et al. 2009.

cutaneous scleroderma are more likely to have progressive disease with internal organ involvement and should be monitored closely. Autoantibody detection may be helpful in the diagnosis and prognostication of disease progression. The treatment is directed at the most symptomatic clinical manifestations, but early aggressive therapy may be organ-sparing, such as the utilization of ACE inhibitors in renal disease and mild hypertension and cytotoxic therapy in interstitial lung disease. Aggressive new treatments being investigated include stem cell transplantation as well as early use of imatinib.

IDIOPATHIC INFLAMMATORY MYOSITIS

Idiopathic inflammatory myopathies are rare acquired disorders characterized by muscle inflammation and weakness. The three recognized types of idiopathic inflammatory myopathies are dermatomyositis, polymyositis, and sporadic inclusion body myositis. These inflammatory myopathies are distinct based on clinical presentation, histopathology, and serologic assessment. In this section, we focus on dermatomyositis and polymyositis, which have an estimated annual incidence between 1.9 and 7.7 per 1 million. Two additional subgroups of inflammatory myositis that will be discussed in this chapter include antisynthetase syndrome and amyopathic dermatomyositis; the annual incidences for these two disorders have not been well defined due to their rarity. Dermatomyositis occurs in any age group, including children, whereas polymyositis typically presents after the second decade of life. Like many autoimmune disorders, dermatomyositis and polymyositis are more common among females, with a female-to-male ratio of 2:1. Idiopathic inflammatory myopathies have been described in association with other autoimmune processes, such as scleroderma and connective tissue disease.

Differential Diagnosis

Idiopathic inflammatory myositis should be distinguished from other myopathic disease processes. The differential diagnosis for myopathy is provided in **Table 14.6**. This table offers a broad differential for myopathies but is not fully inconclusive of all potential etiologies. Idiopathic inflammatory myopathy is characterized by autoimmune related inflammation and can be differentiated from other myopathies by clinical history, examination, and studies such as electromyography (EMG) and muscle biopsy, which are discussed later in this chapter.

Table 14.6   Differential Diagnosis of Myopathy[9]

Idiopathic inflammatory myopathy
- Polymyositis
- Dermatomyositis
- Sporadic inclusion body myositis

Toxin/drug-induced myopathy
- Statins
- Steroids
- Other myotoxic drugs

(continues)

Table 14.6   Differential Diagnosis of Myopathy,[9] cont'd

Endocrine-associated myopathy
- Hypothyroidism
- Hyperthyroidism
- Cortisol excess

Infections
- Lyme
- HIV
- Viral syndromes

Neurogenic disease
- Myasthenia gravis
- Eaton-Lambert syndrome

Muscular dystrophies
- Duchenne's
- Becket's

Metabolic myopathies
- Disorders of glycogen metabolism
- Disorders of lipid metabolism
- Mitochondrial myopathies

Adapted from Burr et al, 2008.

Clinical Features

Both dermatomyositis and polymyositis typically present with the development of proximal muscle weakness over weeks to months. A major clinical feature distinguishing dermatomyositis and polymositis is the presence or lack of cutaneous involvement, respectively. Characteristic skin manifestations in dermatomyositis include a heliotrope rash, a violaceous rash involving the periorbital region; the shawl sign, an erythematous rash over the back and shoulders; the V-sign, an erythematous rash appearing on the face, neck, and anterior chest in described pattern; and Gottron's papules, which are violaceous rash or papules on the metacarpaphalangeal and interphalangeal joints. Additional cutaneous involvement includes periungual dilated capillary loops and subcutaneous calcifications. Antisynthetase syndrome often presents with dermatomyositis-like features, as well as arthritis, idiopathic interstitial lung disease, and Raynaud's phenomenon. In addition, patients affected with antisynthetase syndrome may demonstrate on clinical examination features described as "mechanic's hand," where the palmar aspect of the fingers appears rough and cracked with linear fissures. Amyopathic dermatomyositis is diagnosed in patients who present with cutaneous manifestations consistent with dermatomyositis but who do not exhibit muscle weakness on exam; however, there may be muscle inflammation noted by EMG studies or muscle biopsy. A synopsis of these inflammatory myopathies' characteristic findings is described in **Table 14.7.**

Table 14.7   Idiopathic Inflammatory Myositis Clinical Features[10]

Feature	Polymyositis	Dermatomyositis	Amyopathic Dermatomyositis	Antisynthetase Syndrome
Age of onset	>18 yrs	All ages	>18 yrs	>18 yrs
Proximal weakness	Present	Present	Absent	Typically present
Skin manifestations	Absent	Present	Present	Absent/Present
EMG	Myopathy	Myopathy	Nonspecific of myopathy	Myopathy
Muscle biopsy	Muscle inflammation, CD8/MHC1 complex present	Perivascular and perifascicular inflammation, CD4 and B-Cell infiltration	Nonspecific or pattern consistent with dermatomyositis	Nonspecific or pattern consistent with either polymyositis or dermatomyositis
Muscle enzyme	Elevated	Elevated	Normal or elevated	Elevated

Adapted from Dalakas et al., 2003.

Both polymyositis and dermatomyositis may also present with extraskeletal muscular manifestations involving the gastrointestinal tract and cardiopulmonary system. Gastrointestinal disease can present with dysphagia due to oropharyngeal weakness. Cardiac manifestations include arrhythmias and myocarditis.

Pulmonary involvement can be devastating in patients with inflammatory myositis. Manifestations of pulmonary disease include respiratory muscle weakness, increased risk for aspiration pneumonia, and idiopathic interstitial lung disease. Interstitial lung disease occurs in 60 to 70% of patients with polymyositis and dermatomyositis. Although most interstitial lung disease associated with idiopathic inflammatory myositis are mild and chronic in nature, patients that present with acute interstitial lung disease manifested with a forced vital capacity of less than 65%, diffuse alveolar damage, and amyopathic dermatomyositis features have a very poor prognosis.

An increased risk for malignancy has also been characterized for patients with dermatomyositis and polymyositis. Malignancies have been found preceding, following, and at time of diagnosis. The most common cancers that have been diagnosed in association with inflammatory myositis include gastrointestinal, breast, lung, ovarian, and hematologic malignancies. It has been reported that successful malignancy treatment has resulted in remission of the idiopathic inflammatory myopathy. Given this, patients with inflammatory myositis should be routinely screened for malignancy.

Diagnosis

Diagnosis of inflammatory myositis is based not only on the clinical features just described, but also by additional studies involving muscle analysis and serologic studies. Muscle studies include EMG studies, muscle imaging by magnetic resonance imaging (MRI), and tissue biopsy. Both EMG and MRI are helpful in evaluating for muscle inflammation and localizing an area for tissue biopsy. The myopathic pattern on EMG is characterized by spontaneous activity with decreased amplitude and duration, but it is nonspecific for inflammatory myositis. MRI by either T2-weighted imagery or short tau inversion recovery (STIR) imagery is utilized to eliminate the fat signal and enhance detection of muscle edema, which appears as a hyperintense signal that occurs with muscle inflammation. MRI has several advantages over EMG; it is less invasive, avoids technician variability, and can be used to monitor for disease activity over time with comparison images.

Muscle biopsy allows for histologic diagnosis for either dermatomyositis or polymyositis. Perivascular inflammation and inflammation around the muscle fiber fascicles with perifascicular atrophy is characteristic of dermatomyositis. Lymphocytic infiltration of the perivascular inflammation in dermatomyositis is typically composed of B lymphocytes and CD4-positive T cells. In contrast, inflammation is seen within the muscle fibers of individuals affected with polymyositis. Interestingly, lymphocytic infiltration in polymyositis is characterized by CD8-positive T cells. A second muscle biopsy may be required to increase diagnostic sensitivity.

Laboratory studies utilized in diagnosis of polymyositis and dermatomyositis include biochemical analysis of serum enzymes related to muscle inflammation and detection of associated autoimmune antibodies. The most common serum enzyme measured in idiopathic inflammatory myositis is creatine kinase (CK). CK levels are typically elevated as high as 50-fold greater than normal, but levels do not always correlate with disease activity. In addition, CK levels may be normal with subclinical disease. Other serum enzymes that may be elevated in polymyositis and dermatomyositis include aldolase, lactate dehydrogenase, aspartate aminotransferase, and alanine transferase. Elevations in these serum enzymes are less specific for disease activity.

Identification of autoimmune antibodies related to polymyositis and dermatomyositis is an active and growing field. These autoantibodies are separated into two categories, myositis-specific antibodies (MSA) and myositis-associated antibodies (MAA). Myositis-associated antibodies are present in other autoimmune disorders, such as connective tissue disease. Only about 25% of patients diagnosed with idiopathic inflammatory myositis have positive serologies for currently known MSA, which suggests that there are other MSA yet to be identified. The linkage between various known MSA with clinical manifestations and disease mechanism of inflammatory myositis is still an ongoing investigation. Most MSA are directed against antigens involved in protein synthesis and maturation. More recently identified MSA target nuclear antigens involved in DNA regulation and repair. **Table 14.8** lists the most well-characterized MSA and targets. In addition to those listed, a host of newly recognized MSA are currently being characterized, and identifying novel MSA is an active area of investigation.

Table 14.8   Myositis-Specific Autoantibodies (MSA)[10–13]

MSA	Antigen	Antigen Function	MSA Frequency	Clinical Phenotype
Anti-aminoacyl-tRNA synthetases	tRNA synthetases	Protein synthesis		Antisynthetase syndrome
Anti-Jo1	Histidyl		~20%	
Anti-PL-7	Threonyl			
Anti-PL-12	Alanyl			
Anti-EJ	Glycyl			
Anti-OJ	Isoleucyl			
Anti-KS	Asparagyl			
Anti-SRP	Signal recognition particle	RNP complex involved in protein translocation	~5%	Polymyositis associated with treatment refractory
Anti-Mi2	Mi2	Nuclear helicase involved in gene transcription	~10%	Dermatomyositis associated with treatment responsiveness

Adapted from Gunawardena et al., 2008 & 2009, Hengstman et al., 2001, and Dalakas et al., 2003.

Pathogenesis

The exact autoimmune-mediated mechanism leading to polymyositis and dermatomyositis is still undefined. Factors such as hormones, genes, and environment are believed to play a role in susceptibility to disease development. MSA may play a role in driving autoimmune-mediated inflammation. Histopathology of affected muscles has provided some clues that the pathogenesis between polymyositis and dermatomyositis differ. In polymyositis, muscle fibers express major histocompatibility complex class I (MHC-I) and occasionally MHC complex class II (MHC-II). Muscle fibers do not typically express MHC, and the mechanism leading to the expression of MHC remains unclear. However, the expression of MHC-I provides antigenic presentation for T cell recognition, primarily CD8 cells. In contrast, complement activation leading to recruitment of B lymphocyte and CD4 cells is believed to play a role in the development of dermatomyositis. The autoimmune pathway leading to idiopathic inflammatory myopathy and different clinical manifestations remains an active area of investigation.

Treatment

Steroids are the first-line therapy in idiopathic inflammatory myopathy. Affected individuals typically require high-dose steroid therapy (prednisone, 1 mg/kg/day) and occasionally intravenous pulse-dose steroid therapy is started if myositis is life-threatening. Following high-dose therapy, steroid use is tapered slowly over weeks to months and the taper is guided primarily by clinical response. Changes in CK and other biochemical studies may not correlate with clinical response. Steroid-sparing immunosuppressive agents may need to be added either due to incomplete response to the steroid itself or to aid in tapering the steroid due to steroid-related toxicity. Immunomodulators that have been utilized for idiopathic inflammatory myopathies include azathioprine, methotrexate, cyclosporine, mycophenolate mofetil, and cyclophosamide. Alternative therapies, such as intravenous immunoglobulin, have also been used with promising effect. Investigations into whether biologics, such as TNF-blockers and rituximab, may be effective in idiopathic inflammatory myopathy are currently underway.

In addition to immunosuppressive therapy, patients with idiopathic inflammatory myopathies have other management issues. Some of these management issues are directed at improving patient strength and quality of life, whereas others are focused on addressing the other potential clinical manifestations of inflammatory myopathies or toxicity of medical therapy. Although in the past patients with inflammatory myositis were discouraged from exercising due to concerns for increasing muscle inflammation, recent studies have changed this perspective and practice. Although none of these studies are large-scale, most outcome-benefit studies have demonstrated positive results in muscle strength and endurance without exacerbating muscle inflammation from resistance and aerobic exercise routines under guidance of a physical therapist. Similarly, patients affected by oropharyngeal weakness may benefit from evaluation by a speech therapist to learn techniques to avoid aspiration. In extreme cases of dysphagia, where aspiration is high risk, patients may need to obtain nutritional intake temporarily by tube feeding until oropharyngeal strength is regained.

As noted earlier, pulmonary complications can occur in idiopathic inflammatory myopathy, not only by damage caused by aspiration from oropharyngeal weakness, but also by respiratory muscle weakness and the development of idiopathic interstitial lung disease. Patients may be asymptomatic at the time of diagnosis but still have evidence for pulmonary disease. Given this, patients newly diagnosed with polymyositis and dermatomyositis should be screened for pulmonary disease by pulmonary function tests and radiographic examinations. If initial pulmonary function tests and chest radiography have abnormalities, high-resolution computed tomography (CT) scans should be obtained to characterize idiopathic interstitial lung disease. The frequency of pulmonary evaluation, quarterly versus yearly, for affected individuals has not been well defined. Additionally, patients who may not have pulmonary disease at initial diagnosis should be routinely monitored for development of pulmonary involvement, particularly if they develop new pulmonary symptoms such as shortness of breath or cough.

Polymyositis and dermatomyositis are associated with malignancies; therefore screening for malignancy at time of diagnosis and routinely in follow-up has been recommended. However, no specific guidelines are available due to the wide variety of malignancies that have been found in association with polymyositis and dermatomyositis. A reasonable approach is performing routine age-appropriate screening for malignancies at time of diagnosis and in follow-up. In addition, women diagnosed with an idiopathic inflammatory myopathy may consider having their ovaries imaged to rule out ovarian cancer. Some practitioners may recommend whole-body imaging at the time of diagnosis to localize occult tumors, but the risks and benefits of radiographic exposure should be considered. Although most cases of malignancy found in association with idiopathic inflammatory myopathies occur within the first 5 years of diagnosis, malignancy may appear as late as 20 years after the initial diagnosis. Given this, a high clinical suspicion and awareness for underlying malignancy should be remembered when caring for patients with idiopathic inflammatory myopathies.

Due to exposure from high-dose steroids and possible additional immunosuppressive therapy, patients with idiopathic inflammatory myopathy are susceptible to bone loss and pneumocystis pneumonia. Patients on therapy should have routine bone density tests and be initiated on calcium with vitamin D supplementation as well as bisphosphonates. Exercise regimens, as noted earlier, also help with preventing bone loss and maintaining balance and agility to prevent fractures from mechanical falls. Lastly, prophylaxis against infection by *Pneumocystis jirovecii* is beneficial for patients with idiopathic inflammatory myopathy. Prophylaxis choices include sulfamethoxazole/trimethroprim, pentamidine inhalation, or atovaquone.

Prognosis

Patients with dermatomyositis and polymyositis have an increased risk of death compared to the general population. The mortality risk ranges, on average, between 20 to 70% at 5 years and 40 to 75% at 10 years between various studies. Variability is likely due to study size, delay in diagnosis, and therapeutic management. In the adult population, clinical remission off immunosuppressive drugs is a rarity. Most adults with dermatomyositis or polymyositis, up to 80% in one study, have a chronic or polycyclic course requiring long-term immunosuppressive therapy. In contrast, juvenile dermatomyositis has a better prognosis if aggressive treatment is undertaken without delay. Although an average of 20% of adult patients with idiopathic inflammatory myopathy obtain remission, studies on juvenile dermatomyositis report a higher percentage of possible remission, as high as 58% in one study. Factors associated with increased mortality and morbidity include presence of antisynthetase antibody, advanced age, male sex, and complications related to malignancy and/or pulmonary disease in association with idiopathic inflammatory myopathy.

Summary

Idiopathic inflammatory myopathy is a group of autoimmune-mediated diseases that lead not only to muscle inflammation, but also to other systemic clinical manifestations, such as idiopathic interstitial lung disease, which can be devastating. Idiopathic inflammatory myopathy should be differentiated from other causes of myopathy. Clinical history and examination, as well as studies on muscle tissue and serologic analysis aid in the diagnosis of polymyositis and dermatomyositis. Active investigation identifying MSA and their role in the pathogenesis as well as other autoimmune-mediated pathways will help define future methods of diagnosis, prognosticate disease course, and guide treatment.

SJOGREN'S SYNDROME

Sjogren's syndrome is an autoimmune disorder characterized by lymphocytic infiltration into target organs, typically exocrine glands. Sjogren's syndrome can manifest alone as a primary syndrome or occur in association with other rheumatic conditions, such as rheumatoid arthritis, systemic lupus, or progressive systemic sclerosis. Sjogren's syndrome affects between 0.5 and 2% of the population. It is more common in females, with a female-to-male ratio of 9:1. The syndrome affects all age groups. In women, the syndrome peaks after menarche and after menopause, suggesting that hormonal factors contribute to the disorder's etiology.

Pathogenesis

The exact mechanism leading to Sjogren's syndrome has not been definitively characterized and/or defined. The histopathology from targeted organs such as the salivary gland typically shows lymphocytic infiltration, predominantly T cells, with a CD4-to-CD8 ratio of 3:1 to 5:1. B cells compose 20% of the lymphocytic infiltration and demonstrate hyperreactivity with increased production of autoantibodies and gamma globulins. The interplay between T cells and B cells leading to inflammation of glandular epithelial cells continues to be investigated. In addition to altered immune responses, current research also focuses on the pathogenic contributions of genetic, hormonal, and autonomic factors.

Diagnosis

In 2002, an International American–European Study Group was formed to examine prior Sjogren's syndrome classification criteria, which were formed and validated in 1989 and 1996 by the European Study Group on Classification Criteria for Sjogren's Syndrome.

From the American–European Study Group, a revised version of the Classification Criteria for Sjogren's syndrome was developed (**Table 14.9**).

Table 14.9   Revised International Classification Criteria for Sjogren's Syndrome[14]

Ocular symptoms (must attest to at least one ocular symptom)
  a. Daily, persistent troublesome dry eyes for more than 3 months
  b. Recurrent sensation of sand or gravel in the eyes
  c. Use of tear of substitutes more than three times a day

Oral symptoms (must attest to at least one oral symptom)
  a. Daily feeling of dry mouth for more than 3 months
  b. Recurrent or persistent swollen salivary glands as an adult
  c. Frequently requires drinking liquid to aid in swallowing dry food

Objective signs of lacrimal involvement (must have one objective finding)
  a. Schirmer's test: if less than 5 mm of filter paper is wetted after 5 minutes from the lower conjunctival sac
  b. Rose bengal score greater than 4 by the von Bijsterveld scoring system

Objective signs of salivary gland involvement (must have one objective finding)
  a. Sialometry measuring less than 1.5 ml of unstimulated salivary flow into calibrated tube for 15 minutes
  b. Parotid sialography showing abnormal pattern of parotid ductules without evidence of gross obstruction in major ducts
  c. Salivary gland scintigraphy demonstrating delayed uptake or excretion of technetium Tc 99m pertechnetate

Histopathology of minor salivary gland
  Evidence of greater than one foci of focal lymphocytic sialadenitis, which is defined by 50 or more lymphocytes surrounding vascular or ductal areas, per 4 mm^2 of glandular tissue

Autoantibody
  Having one or both antibodies to Ro (SSA) and La (SSB) in the serum

Adapted from Vitali et al., 2002.

Diagnosis for primary Sjogren's syndrome is met if four of the six criteria in Table 14.9 are present, as long as one of the criteria is either a positive histopathology of the minor salivary gland or presence of serum autoantibody. Alternatively, a patient may be classified as having primary Sjogren's syndrome if three of four objective criteria are present. Secondary Sjogren's syndrome is diagnosed in patients who have a known rheumatic disease, such as rheumatoid arthritis or other defined connective tissue disease, and either ocular or oral symptoms and two of the objective findings in Table 14.9. Patients are excluded from the diagnosis of primary Sjogren's syndrome if they have a history of head and neck radiation treatment, active infection with viruses such as hepatitis C and HIV, sarcoidosis, preexisting lymphoma, graft-versus-host disease, or anticholinergic drugs use. The revised international classification criteria for Sjogren's syndrome have a sensitivity and specificity of 96.1% and 94.2%, respectively.

Clinical Manifestation

Sjogren's syndrome typically involves the exocrine glands of the eyes and mouth with clinical symptoms of dry eyes, dry mouth, and swollen parotid glands. Up to one-third of patients will have extraglandular manifestations. Both glandular and extraglandular clinical manifestations are described in **Table 14.10**.

Table 14.10   Clinical Manifestations of Sjogren's Syndrome[15,16]

Organ System	Signs/Symptoms
Ocular	Xerophthalmia, keratoconjunctivitis, blepharitis, iritis, uveitis
Oral	Xerostomia, periodontal disease, oral candidiasis, sialadenitis
Musculoskeletal	Arthralgia, arthritis
Skin	Xerosis, Raynaud's syndrome, cutaneous vasculitis
Pulmonary	Xerotrachea, interstitial lung disease (nonspecific pneumonitis, bronchiolitis obliterans and organizing pneumonia, usual interstitial pneumonitis, lymphocytic interstitial pneumonitis), pulmonary hypertension
Gastrointestinal	Gastritis, esophageal and gastric dysmotility, pancreatitis, hepatitis
Renal	Tubulointerstitial nephritis, interstitial cystitis, renal vasculitis
Neurologic	Cranial neuropathies, peripheral neuropathies (sensory more common), sensorineural hearing loss
Hematologic	Lymphoma

Adapted from Fox 2005 and Kassan et al., 2004.

Of note, patients with Sjogren's syndrome have a 40-fold increased risk of developing lymphoma. Clinical signs suggestive of the development of lymphoma include persistent parotid gland enlargement, lymphadenopathy, splenomegaly, and evidence of vasculitis, such as palpable purpura and nonhealing leg ulcers. Serologic markers of concern for the development of lymphoma in patients affected with Sjogren's syndrome include hypergammaglobulinemia, mixed monoclonal cryoglobulinemia, and low levels of complement C4.

Treatment

The treatment of Sjogren's syndrome is symptomatic. Sicca symptoms, such as xeropthalmia and xerostomia, are treated with moisture replacement therapy and secretagogues, pilocarpine and cevimeline, which stimulate the muscarinic receptor. Xerostomia increases the risk for dental caries, and vigilant dental care in patients with Sjogren's syndrome is necessary to prevent periodontal disease as well as secondary complications such as oral candidiasis. The treatment of extraglandular manifestations of Sjogren's syndrome is less well studied. Corticosteroids, NSAIDs, and hydroxychloroquine have all been utilized in Sjogren's syndrome patients for treating nonvisceral disease, such as arthritis, but the overall effectiveness of these medications by clinical studies has not been measured. Similar to systemic sclerosis, treatment of Raynaud's phenomena in Sjogren's syndrome include keeping distal extremities warm to utilization of dihidropiridine-type calcium antagonists to optimize vascular perfusion. In extreme cases where digital ulceration is at risk, treatment with intravenous prostanoids, bosentan, and sildanefil may be considered. Likewise, bosentan, sitaxentin, and/or sildanefil may be used to control pulmonary hypertension secondary to Sjogren's syndrome. The treatment for the extraglandular manifestations of Sjogren's syndrome, including nephritis, interstitial lung damage, neuropathy, and vasculitis, has not been well defined. Steroid-sparing immunomodulator agents, such as azathioprine and methotrexate; cytotoxic drugs, such as cyclophosphamide; and biologic therapy, such as tumor necrosis factor inhibitors have been utilized as treatments in non-randomized studies and case reports.

RELAPSING POLYCHONDRITIS

Relapsing polychondritis is a rare autoimmune disorder characterized by recurrent inflammation of cartilaginous tissue. The incidence has been estimated to be 3.5 cases per 1 million. Most case series report the incidence as being equal between male and females; however, one series had a female-to-male ratio of 3:1. Relapsing polychondritis has been diagnosed in all age groups, but the mean age of onset is between the fourth and fifth decade of life.

Diagnosis

Relapsing polychondritis is difficult to diagnose because there is no specific diagnostic test. The diagnostic criteria first proposed by McAdam et al.[17] in 1979 have since been modified. These criteria are focused on the clinical manifestations of relapsing polychondritis, as noted in **Table 14.11**.

Table 14.11   Diagnostic Criteria for Relapsing Polychondritis[17]

Chondritis
a. Auricular, typically bilateral and sparing inferior lobule
b. Nasal
c. Laryngotracheal
Ocular inflammation
Audiovestibular damage
Inflammatory arthritis

Adapted from McAdam et al., 1979.

Diagnostic criteria are met if chondritis is present at two sites or if chondritis is present at one site with two of the three additional clinical manifestations. If only one ear is inflamed, infection should be considered in the differential diagnosis. When inflammation with structural damage is present at the nasal and laryngotracheal region, the differential diagnosis should also include ANCA-associated vasculitis and sarcoidosis, as well as infections such as tuberculosis, leprosy, and syphilis.

Clinical Manifestations

Although inflammation of cartilaginous tissue is a primary feature of relapsing polychondritis, it is a systemic disease affecting many organ systems. The clinical manifestations are provided in **Table 14.12**.

Table 14.12   Clinical Manifestations of Relapsing Polychondritis[18,19]

Organ System	Signs/Symptoms
Cartilage	Auricular chondritis, nasal chondritis, laryngotracheal chondritis
Ocular	Episcleritis, scleritis, xeropthalmia, keratoconjunctivitis, iritis, retinopathy, keratitis, and optic neuritis
Musculoskeletal	Arthritis—typically seronegative, nonerosive, intermittent, migratory, and asymmetric
Skin	Leukocytoclastic vasculitis, septal panniculitis, ulcerations, distal necrosis
Mucosal	Oral ulcers, genital ulcers
Pulmonary	Tracheobronchial stenosis, obstructive bronchietasis
Cardiovascular	Aortic/mitral regurgitation, aortitis, aortic aneurysm (thoracic and abdominal), pericarditis, conduction abnormalities, thrombosis (arterial and venous)
Renal	Tubulointerstitial nephritis, mesangial expansion, IgA nephropathy, segmental necrotizing crescentic glomerulonephritis
Neurologic	Cranial neuropathies, headaches, seizures, rhomboencephalitis

Created with information from Kent et al, 2004 and Trentham et al, 1998.

Due to the recurring and relapsing inflammation of cartilaginous tissue, deformities can occur, leading to secondary complications. With auricular chondritis, "cauliflower" deformity may develop. Conductive hearing loss may also occur. Saddle deformity may occur as a structural complication from nasal chondritis. Repeated laryngotracheal inflammation may result in vocal cord palsy and laryngotracheal stenosis or collapse. Patients with relapsing polychondritis should have regular pulmonary function tests to measure for signs of airway compromise.

In addition to the list of potential clinical manifestations related to relapsing polychondritis noted in Table 14.12, relapsing polychondritis has also been found in association with other diseases. It has been associated with other autoimmune disorders, including systemic vasculitides, such as ANCA-associated vasculitis and Behcet's, as well as connective tissue diseases, such as rheumatoid arthritis and systemic lupus erythematosus. Relapsing polychondritis has been associated with endocrine disorders such as autoimmune thyroid disorders and diabetes, as well as thymoma. In addition, it has been associated with inflammatory bowel diseases. Lastly, relapsing polychondritis is associated with hematologic malignancies, predominantly myelodysplastic syndrome. Patient with relapsing polychondritis presenting with skin manifestations and findings suggestive of vasculitis should be assessed for underlying malignancy.

Pathogenesis

The mechanism of disease leading to relapsing polychondritis is not known. Antibodies to collagen types II, IX, and XI have been identified, but their association to the disease itself is unclear. There is some increased association of relapsing polychondritis in patients carrying human leukocyte antigen (HLA)-DR4 and a negative association with HLA-DR6. How these factors contribute to the pathogenesis of relapsing polychondritis has yet to be determined.

Treatment

Like many autoimmune disorders, the main form of therapy for relapsing polychondritis is oral corticosteroids. Low-dose corticosteroid therapy may be sufficient for mild disease, but high-dose therapy is required for disease with systemic involvement and risks of end organ damage. Additional medications that have been reported for management of relapsing polychondritis include NSAIDs and colchicine. Steroid-sparing agents and/or cytotoxic agents can be utilized for visceral disease but effectiveness has not been evaluated in clinical trials.

◇◇◇◇◇◇◇◇◇◇◇◇

REFERENCES

1. Foti R, Leonardi R, Rondinone R, et al. Scleroderma-like disorders. *Autoimmunity Rev.* 2008;7:331–339.

2. Masi AT, Rodnan GP, Medsger TA, et al. Subcommittee for scleroderma criteria of the American Rheumatism Association Diagnostic and Therapeutic Criteria Committee. Preliminary criteria for the classification of systemic sclerosis (Scleroderma). *Arthritis Rheum.* 1980;23:581–590.

3. Walker JG, Pope J, Baron M, et al. The development of systemic sclerosis classification criteria. *Clin Rheumatol.* 2007;26:1401–1409.

4. Shah AA, Wigley FM. Often forgotten manifestations of systemic sclerosis. *Rheum Dis Clin N Am.* 2008;34:221–238.

5. Steen VD. The many faces of scleroderma. *Rheum Dis Clin N Am.* 2008;34:1–15.

6. Gabrielli A, Avvedimento EV, Krieg T. Scleroderma: mechanisms of disease. *N Engl J Med.* 2009;360:1989–2003.

7. Harris ML, Rosen A. Autoimmunity in scleroderma: the origin, pathogenetic role, and clinical significance of autoantibodies. *Curr Opin Rheumatol.* 2003; 15:778–784.

8. Kowal-Bielecka O, Landewe R, Avouac J, et al. EULAR recommendations for the treatment of systemic sclerosis: a report from the EULAR Scleroderma Trials and Research group (EUSTAR). *Ann Rheum Dis.* 2009;68:620–628.

9. Burr ML, Roos JC, Oster AJK. Metabolic myopathies: a guide and update for clinicians. *Curr Opin Rheumatol.* 2008;20:639–647.

10. Dalakas MC, Hohlfeld R. Polymyositis and dermatomyositis. *Lancet.* 2003; 362: 971–982.

11. Gunawardena H, Betteridge ZE, McHugh NJ. Newly identified autoantibodies: relationship to idiopathic inflammatory myopathy subsets and pathogenesis. *Curr Opin Rheumatol.* 2008;20:675–680.

12. Gunawardena H, Betteridge ZE, and McHugh NJ. Myositis-specific autoantibodies: their clinical and pathogenic significance in disease expression. *Rheumatology.* 2009;48:607–612.

13. Hengstman GJD, van Engelen BGM, Vree Egberts WTM, et al. Myositis-specific autoantibodies: overview and recent developments. *Curr Opin Rheumatol.* 2001;13:476–482.

14. Vitali C, Bombardieri S, Jonsson R, et al. Classification criteria for Sjogren's syndrome: a revised version of the European criteria proposed by the American-European Consensus Group. *Ann Rheum Dis.* 2002;61:554–558.

15. Fox RI. Sjogren's Syndrome. *Lancet.* 2005;366:321–331.

16. Kassan SS, Moutsopoulos HM. Clinical Manifestations and early diagnosis of Sjogren's syndrome. *Arch Intern Med.* 2004;164:1275–1284.

17. McAdam LP, O'Hanlan MA, Bluestone R, et al. Relapsing polychondritis: prospective study of 23 patients and a review of the literature. *Medicine (Baltimore).* 1976;55:193–215.

18. Kent PD, Michet CJ, Luthra HS. Relapsing polychondritis. *Curr Opin Rheumatol.* 2004;16:56–61.

19. Trentham DE, Le CH. Relapsing polychondritis. *Ann Intern Med.* 1998;129:114–122.

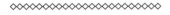

SUGGESTED READINGS

SCLERODERMA

Allanore Y, Meune C, Kahan A. Systemic sclerosis and cardiac dysfunction: evolving concepts and diagnostic methodologies. *Curr Opin Rheumatol.* 2008;20:697–702.

Antoniou KM, Wells AU. Scleroderma lung disease: evolving understanding in light of newer studies. *Curr Opin Rheumatol.* 2008;20:686–691.

Avouac J, Kowal-Bielecka O, Landewe R, et al. European League Against Rheumatism (EULAR) Scleroderma Trial and Research group (EUSTAR) recommendations for the treatment of systemic sclerosis: methods of elaboration and results of systematic literature research. *Ann Rheum Dis.* 2009;68:629–634.

Czirjak L, Foeldvari I, Muller-Ladner U. Skin involvement in systemic sclerosis. *Rheumatology.* 2008;47:v44–v45.

Doran JP, Veale DJ. Biomarkers in systemic sclerosis. *Rheumatology.* 2008; 47:v36–v38.

Leroy EC, Black C, Fleischmajer R, et al. Scleroderma (systemic sclerosis): classification, subsets, and pathogenesis. *J. Rheumatology.* 1988;15:202–205.

Penn H, Denton CP. Diagnosis, management and prevention of scleroderma renal disease. *Curr Opin Rheumatol.* 2008;20:692–696.

IDIOPATHIC INFLAMMATORY MYOSITIS

Airio A, Kautiainen H, Hakala M. Prognosis and mortality of polymyositis and dermatomyositis patients. *Clin Rheumatol.* 2006;25:234–239.

Alexanderson, H. Exercise effects in patients with adult idiopathic inflammatory myopathies. *Curr Opin Rheumatol.* 2009;21:158–163.

Bronner IM, van der Meulen MFG, de Visser M, et al. Long-term outcome in polymyositis and dermatomyositis. *Ann Rheum Dis.* 2006;65:1456–1461.

Burr ML, Roos JC, Oster AJ. Metabolic myopathies: a guide and update for clinicians. *Curr Opin Rheumatol.* 2008;20:639–647.

Choy EHS, Isenberg DA. Treatment of dermatomyositis and polymyositis. *Rheumatology.* 2002;41:7–13.

Dalakas MC, Hohlfeld R. Polymyositis and dermatomyositis. *Lancet.* 2003;362:971–982.

Dayal NA, Isenberg DA. Assessment of inflammatory myositis. *Curr Opin Rheumatol.* 2001;13:488–492.

Fathi M, Vikgren J, Boijsen M, et al. Interstitial lung disease in polymyositis and dermatomyositis: longitudinal evaluation by pulmonary function and radiology. *Arth Care Res.* 2008;59:677–685.

Gunawardena H, Betteridge ZE, McHugh NJ. Newly identified autoantibodies: relationship to idiopathic inflammatory myopathy subsets and pathogenesis. *Curr Opin Rheumatol.* 2008;20:675–680.

Gunawardena H, Betteridge ZE, and McHugh NJ. Myositis-specific autoantibodies: their clinical and pathogenic significance in disease expression. *Rheumatology.* 2009;48:607–612.

Hengstman GJD, van Engelen BGM, Vree Egberts WTM, et al. Myositis-specific autoantibodies: overview and recent developments. *Curr Opin Rheumatol.* 2001;13:476–482.

Kang EH, Lee EB, Shin KC, et al. Interstitial lung disease in patients with polymyositis, dermatomyositis and amyopathic dermatomyositis. *Rheumatology.* 2005;44:1282–1286.

Kim S, El-Hallak M, Dedeoglu F, et al. Complete and sustained remission of juvenile dermatomyositis resulting from aggressive treatment. *Arthritis Rheum.* 2009;60:1825–1830.

Maoz CR, Langevitz P, Livneh A, et al. High Incidence of malignancies in patients with dermatomyositis and polymyositis: an 11-year analysis. *Semin Arthritis Rheum.* 1998;27:319–324.

Tomasova Studynkova J, Charvat F, Jarosova K, et al. The role of MRI in the assessment of polymyositis and dermatomyositis. *Rheumatology.* 2007;46:1174–1179.

Walker UA. Imaging tools for the clinical assessment of idiopathic inflammatory myositis. *Curr Opin Rheumatol.* 2008;20:656–661.

SJOGREN'S SYNDROME

Bowman SJ, Sutcliffe N, Isenberg DA, et al. Sjogren's Systemic Clinical Activity Index (SCAI)—a systemic disease activity measure for use in clinical trial in primary Sjogren's syndrome. *Rheumatology.* 2007;46:1845–1851.

Fox RI. Sjogren's syndrome. *Lancet.* 2005; 366:321–331.

Hansen A, Lipsky PE, Dorner T. Immunopathogenesis of primary Sjogren's syndrome: implications for disease management and therapy. *Curr Opin Rheumatol.* 2005;17:558–565.

Kassan SS, Moutsopoulos HM. Clinical manifestations and early diagnosis of Sjogren's syndrome. *Arch Intern Med.* 2004;164:1275–1284.

Mackay F, Groom JR, Tangye SG. An important role for B-cell activation factor and B cells in the pathogenesis of Sjogren's syndrome. *Curr Opin Rheumatol.* 2007;19:406–413.

Ramos-Casals M, Font J. Primary Sjogren's syndrome: current and emergent aetiopathogenic concepts. *Rheumatology.* 2005;44:1354–1367.

Ramos-Casals M, Brito-Zeron P. Emerging biological therapies in primary Sjogren's syndrome. *Rheumatology.* 2007;46:1389–1396.

Vitali C, Bombardieri S, Jonsson R, et al. Classification criteria for Sjogren's syndrome: a revised version of the European criteria proposed by the American-European Consensus Group. *Ann Rheum Dis.* 2002;61:554–558.

RELAPSING POLYCHONDRITIS

Damiani JM, Levin HL. Relapsing polychondritis - report of ten cases. *Laryngoscope.* 1979;89:929–946.

Kent PD, Michet CJ, Luthra HS. Relapsing polychondritis. *Curr Opin Rheumatol.* 2004;16:56–61.

McAdam LP, O'Hanlan MA, Bluestone R, et al. Relapsing polychondritis: prospective study of 23 patients and a review of the literature. *Medicine (Baltimore).* 1976;55:193–215.

Michet CJ, McKenna CH, Luthra HS, et al. Relapsing polychondritis. Survival and predictive role of early disease manifestations. *Ann Intern Med.* 1986;104:74–78.

Trentham DE, Le CH. Relapsing polychondritis. *Ann Intern Med.* 1998;129:114–122.

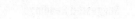

CHAPTER 15

Osteoporosis

Jonathan S. Coblyn, MD
Alan G. Cole, MD

OVERVIEW

Osteoporosis is a disorder of low bone mineral density (BMD) with an associated increased risk for fracture. Most commonly described in postmenopausal women and in older men, it can be seen among younger patients who have predisposing medical conditions, strong family histories, and/or medication exposures. Osteoporosis is defined by bone densitometry, and the diagnosis is based on the finding of a low bone mineral density when compared with population norms of measured peak bone mass at approximately age 30. Given that bone density declines with advancing age and at an increased rate among women as of the onset of menopause, osteoporosis is common and even anticipated among many of the elderly. Two million osteoporosis related fractures had been predicted for 2005, 71% among women, with an associated economic burden of $17 billion.[1] An estimated 300,000 hip fractures occur in the United States yearly attributable to osteoporosis. Hip fracture among the elderly leads to a 50% incidence of permanent disability and a 20% one year excess mortality. Therefore, the importance of osteoporosis and its consequences can hardly be overstated. Some predisposing factors are reversible. In addition, osteoporosis can often be treated or prevented even when it occurs as a result of aging. Therefore given the tools now available, inattention by patients and providers can lead to unnecessary morbidity and mortality. This chapter discusses the etiology and diagnosis of osteoporosis and available treatment options.

DIAGNOSIS

A number of agencies, including the World Health Organization (WHO), have defined osteoporosis as a T-score of bone density < 2.5 standard deviations (SD) below population norm peak adult bone mass (**Table 15.1**). Bone density is reported as a T-score in which the bone density is compared to gender-matched normative values for 30 year olds. BMD is also reported as a Z-score, in which the bone density is compared to normative values of controls matched for current age and gender as well as body weight and ethnicity.

Table 15.1   WHO Definition of Osteoporosis by Bone Mineral Density

Definition	Standard Deviations from "Young Normal Adult"	T-Score
Normal	Within 1	> −1.0
Low bone mass or osteopenia	1.0 to 2.5 below	−1.0 to −2.5
Osteoporosis*	2.5 or above	< −2.5

*Severe osteoporosis is defined as T-score < -2.5 with history of fragility fracture.

Created with information from the World Health Organization Collaborating Centre for Metabolic Bone Diseases, University of Sheffield, UK, 1994 Guidelines

Most specialty professional societies endorse the classification presented in Table 15.1 and further recognize that fracture risk is determined by factors beyond bone density alone. As an example, once an osteoporotic fragility fracture has occurred (i.e. a fracture occurring with minimal trauma, commonly a Colles', hip, or vertebral fracture), fracture risk is such that treatment should be initiated without regard to the patient's WHO category. The most appropriate clinical approach is to define the risk of fracture using bone density along with specific clinical characteristics with use of the FRAX risk calculator (see below) which allows one to make the appropriate treatment decision. Important predisposing factors that promote osteoporosis are noted in **Table 15.2**.

Table 15.2   Risk Factors for Hip Fracture in Women

Risk Factor	Relative Risk
Established Risk Factor	**Relative Risk >2.0**
Bone mineral density	Per 1 SD decrease
Neuromuscular impairment	Unable to rise without arms
History of limited trauma fracture	Suggests increased bone fragility
Age	Increased in age >50
Established Risk Factor	**Relative Risk >1.1–1.9**
Multiple falls	Increased risk
Estrogen replacement therapy	Less risk
Weight	Increased for weight <125
Vision impairment	Increased fall risk
Physical inactivity	Increased if sedentary

(continues)

Table 15.2 Risk Factors for Hip Fracture in Women, cont'd

Risk Factor	Relative Risk
Likely Risk Factors	**Relative Risk >2.0**
Weight loss since age 25	20% loss increases risk
Ethnicity	Increased risk for Caucasians/Asians
Poor health status	Increased risk
Calcium intake <400 mg/day, inadequate vitamin D intake	Increased
Height	Increased with loss of height; taller individuals also at greater risk
Hip axis length	Increased with loss
Sedative use	Increased with use
Smokers (active or passive)	Increased with use

Adapted from Cummings RG, Nevitt MC, Cummings SR. Epidemiology of hip fractures. Epidemiology Rev. 1997;19:244-257, as adapted in: Klippel JH, ed. Primer on the Rheumatic Diseases, 12th Edition. Atlanta, Ga: Arthritis Foundation; 2001.

Often, patients will be suspected of having osteoporosis based on plain radiographs. Plain radiographs may show a bone mineral deficit but are not specific, have low sensitivity and are subject to variations in technique. Only a bone mineral density measurement can reliably diagnose osteoporosis. In turn, bone mineral density measurement will help predict fracture risk and allows one to monitor the effect of therapy. It may also visualize a prior vertebral fracture (**Table 15.3**). The International Society for Clinical Densitometry has developed indications for bone mineral density testing (**Table 15.4**). In addition, because low body weight is associated with low bone density, some experts recommend screening female patients between the ages of 45 and 64 who weigh less than 132 pounds. Note that while a bone density deficit is more common in this subgroup, a finding of osteoporosis in younger individuals should generally be managed differently than in the post-menopausal population (see below).

Table 15.3 Clinical Use of Bone Mineral Density Measurements

- Diagnosis using WHO criteria
- Prediction of fracture risk
- Vertebral fracture assessment
- Monitoring treatment or deciding whether to initiate treatment

Adapted from Miller PD, and Leonard MB. Clinical use of Bone mass measurements in adults for the assessment and management of osteoporosis. In: Favus MJ, ed. Primer on the Metabolic Bone Diseases and Disorders of Mineral Metabolism, 6th Edition. Washington, DC: American Society for Bone and Mineral Research; 2006.

Table 15.4   Clinical Indications for Bone Mass Measurements

- Women aged 65 and older
- Postmenopausal women under age 65 with risk factors
- Men aged 70 and older
- Adults with prior fragility fracture
- Adults with a disease associated with low bone mass or bone loss
- Adults taking medications associated with low bone mass or bone loss
- Any patient being considered for pharmacologic therapy
- Anyone being treated to monitor therapy
- Anyone not receiving treatment in whom evidence of bone loss would lead to treatment

Adapted from Miller PD, and Leonard MB. Clinical use of Bone mass measurements in adults for the assessment and management of osteoporosis. In: Favus MJ, ed. Primer on the Metabolic Bone Diseases and Disorders of Mineral Metabolism, 6th Edition. Washington, DC: American Society for Bone and Mineral Research; 2006.

Many variables must be considered when looking at bone density readings. For example, the measurement can vary by machine (0.5 SD difference). The standard bone density test looks at the hip and spine. Any variation in bone may increase or decrease the measured bone density. The standard bone density test may be of lesser value among patients with spinal deformities, those with osteoarthritis or orthopedic hardware, and those who have had compression deformities. Each of these factors tend to cause spuriously elevated bone density readings. While usual bone density measurements may be unreliable when such interferences are present, one can often obtain clinically useful information from less reliable DXA studies (e.g. omit of one or two affected vertebrae from consideration, perform a lateral spine DXA study to avoid interference from osteophytes, consider a hip study alone when LS spine compression fractures or if there is diffuse osteoarthritis among the lumbar vertebrae). Bone mineral density measurement of the distal ulna and/or the heel can be performed as initial screening tests; they should not be used to follow patients, but can be used to trigger a central study of the hip and spine.

With the advent of more widespread bone mineral density testing, one can now define patients at different risk and thus evolve the diagnosis from normal bone density to osteopenia (SD –1.0 to –2.5) to full-fledged osteoporosis (SD <2.5). The incidence of fracture increases not only as the bone density lessens, but also as age increases. In older patients, there is a higher risk for fragility fractures at similar bone density measurements. In addition, any prior fragility factor increases the risk of further fractures at a given bone density value. At a T-score of –2.5, the incidence of fracture is a little over 10% for a 50-year-old, but increases to almost 35% in an 80-year-old individual.

The single greatest risk factor for osteoporosis is advanced age. Normally, peak bone mass is achieved at age 30 to 35, after which bone mass slowly declines among both men and women. After menopause there is a three-fold increase in the rate of bone density decline. As a result, an early menopause is a prominent promoter of osteoporosis. Additional risk factors for osteoporosis are noted in **Table 15.5** and include the following: Caucasian race; age greater than 50; female gender; family history of osteoporosis;

fracture(s); use of steroids, antiseizure medications and aromatase inhibitors; malabsorption and nutritional deficiency along with endocrine disorders including thyroid and parathyroid disease. Other risk factors include nulliparity, decreased physical activity, alcohol ingestion of ≥3 drinks per day and/or tobacco use. In addition, increased fracture risk may result from decreased muscular function, orthostatic hypotension, cardiac arrhythmia, urinary urgency, poor balance, impaired hearing, sight, or cognition, or from environmental hazards such as use of throw rugs, poor lighting, or slippery outdoor conditions.

Table 15.5   Classification of Osteoporosis/Low Bone Density

Major Type of Osteoporosis	Causative Factors	Details
Primary	Postmenopausal or age-related	
Secondary	Endocrine	Hyperparathyroidism Central amenorrhea (e.g., athletic or nutritional) Hyperthyroidism Type 1 diabetes Cushing's syndrome Acromegaly Hyperprolactinemia Male hypogonadism
	Drugs	Steroids Thyroid hormone Heparin Sedatives, psychotropics Anticonvulsants Cyclosporine Chemotherapy GnRH Aromatase inhibitors
	Hematologic	Multiple myeloma Lymphoma Leukemia Mastocytosis Gaucher's disease
	Rheumatologic	Rheumatoid arthritis Marfan's syndrome Ehlers Danlos
	Congenital	Osteogensis imperfecta
	Immobilization	Including space flight
	Idiopathic hypercalcuria	Renal tubular acidosis

(continues)

Table 15.5   Classification of Osteoporosis/Low Bone Density, cont'd

MAJOR TYPE OF OSTEOPOROSIS	CAUSATIVE FACTORS	DETAILS
Secondary	Renal	Renal osteodystrophy Chronic renal failure
	Pregnancy	Osteoporosis of pregnancy

Adapted from Oxford Handbook of Rheumatology, 2nd edition. Oxford: Oxford University Press, 2006.

Menopause is particularly hard on bone, and approximately 15% of bone mass can be lost within 5 years of menopause. This bone loss is exacerbated by vitamin D deficiency, which is remarkably common in Western society.

Investigation of Osteoporosis

A number of causes of secondary osteoporosis have been identified (**Table 15.5**). Studies are often appropriate and should be performed as guided by clinical assessment (**Table 15.6**). Limited studies should be obtained in virtually all patients with a bone mineral density deficit, including 25-OH vitamin D and serum Ca^{++} levels at a minimum. Vitamin D deficiency is extraordinarily common in the North American population, given the limited sun exposure that many experience, even in the summertime. A limited number of foods contain vitamin D, notably including vitamin D added milk but not dairy products overall. Given that the older half of the population often tends to drink little milk and have limited sun exposure to exposed skin, vitamin D deficiency is quite common in the at-risk population.

While the T-score is a good measure of fracture risk, the Z-score is more useful in determining whether a more thorough investigation for secondary osteoporosis should be undertaken; when ≤1.5, an identifiable cause of osteoporosis beyond age and gender should be pursued. In addition to laboratory studies, a proper history and physical may provide clues. As examples, clinical evidence of hyperthyroidism or malabsorption, prior kidney stones suggesting hypercalciuria, a known anemia (multiple myeloma may cause a diffuse osteoporosis, not necessarily lytic bone lesions), or sexual dysfunction among men may direct one's investigation. Medications may promote osteoporosis, notably steroids (oral, inhaled, nasal, repeated intravenous steroids given during multiple hospitalizations, or multiple doses given by injection for musculoskeletal concerns—see below), seizure medications which increase vitamin D catabolism and therefore vitamin D requirement, or aromatase inhibitors. A history of early menopause or an eating disorder may or may not provide disorder-specific therapy and may add to one's understanding. Hyperparathyroidism is most commonly silent and a PTH and serum Ca^{++} along with TSH, creatinine, SPEP and a 25-OH vitamin D level should be obtained as a minimum when secondary osteoporosis is suspected.

Table 15.6 Laboratory Studies for Diagnostic Screening in Patients with Known Osteoporosis

Complete blood count
Erythrocyte sedimentation rate
Calcium
Phosphate
Albumin
Liver blood studies
Prothrombin time
Creatinine
Alkaline phosphatase
Serum protein electrophoresis
25-OH vitamin D 3 and 1,25 OH vitamin D 3
Urinary calcium and phosphate
Thyroid stimulating hormone
Parathyroid hormone
Dexamethasone suppression test (when appropriate)
Follicle-stimulating hormone, luteinizing hormone, growth hormone (when appropriate)
Vitamin B12
Tissue transglutaminase and other markers of irritable bowel disease/malabsorption

Treatment

The first recommended therapy of osteoporosis is the treatment of an identified cause of reversible secondary osteoporosis. A vitamin D level should be determined among most or all individuals with osteoporosis and the level should be maintained >30–35 ng/ml. When a deficit is present (e.g. a serum level <20 ng/ml), pharmacologic replacement with vitamin D 50,000 IU 1–3 times per week with 8–16 doses given in total. A vitamin D level should be repeated after pharmacologic replacement is completed to ensure adequacy of therapy and a supplement consisting of 1000 IU or more should be recommended afterward on a continuing basis. When a particularly marked vitamin D deficiency is present or when usual pharmacologic replacement is inadequate, confounding circumstances should be considered, e.g. malabsorption or the effect of administered seizure medications.

Under many or most circumstances, reversible secondary osteoporosis is not demonstrated and pharmacologic therapy directed toward increasing bone mineral mass without regard to cause should be considered. A commonly followed set of indications for use of pharmacologic therapy consists of the National Osteoporosis Foundation (NOF) treatment guidelines. Recommendations for the use of approved medication for the treatment of osteoporosis for post-menopausal women and for men ≥age 50 are appropriate under any one of the following circumstances:

- A hip or vertebral (clinical or morphometric) fracture

- T-score ≤2.5 at the femoral neck or spine (after appropriate intervention to treat a reversible secondary cause, e.g. vitamin D deficiency)
- Low bone mass (T-score between –1.0 and –2.5 at the femoral neck or spine) and a 10-year probability of a hip fracture ≥3% or a 10-year probability of a major osteoporosis-related fracture ≥20% based on the US-adapted WHO algorithm
- Clinicians judgment and/or patient preferences may indicate treatment for people with 10-year fracture probabilities above or below these levels

The 10-year fracture probability can be determined with consideration of specific clinical parameters in addition to the bone density measured by DXA. Clinical variables include age, sex, current smoking status, weight and height, alcohol intake, previous fractures, steroid use, diagnosis of rheumatoid arthritis, as well as the femoral neck bone mineral density. The algorithm can be accessed at **www.shef.ac.uk/FRAX**. Observers will note that osteoporosis at any site is considered an indication for therapy in this population without regard to the FRAX calculation, while in the setting of osteopenia, only femoral neck BMD is utilized by the FRAX protocol for risk determination. The FRAX calculation only applies to the post-menopausal (among women) and >age 50 (among men) population. The use of pharmacologic therapy is commonly not advised among individuals <age 50 in the absence of secondary osteoporosis (e.g. chronic steroid administration) because bisphosphonates are not indicated during pregnancy (see below) and, as noted previously, fracture risk is lower at a given bone mineral density among younger individuals.

Supplement Therapy

Adequate calcium intake is recommended for the population-at-large for osteoporosis prevention and therapy and should include 1000 to 1300 mg of elemental calcium (combined dietary and supplement) along with a vitamin D intake of 1000 IU/day or more. In addition, weight-bearing exercise, weight training, and almost any antigravity exercise may have value for prevention and avoidance of progression.

Bisphosphonate Therapy

Currently, four oral and two intravenous bisphosphanate preparations are available. Bisphosphonates decrease bone resorption and have been shown, to different degrees, to alter the fracture risk of the hip and/or of the spine.[5]

Bisphosphonates are the most commonly prescribed pharmacologic agents for the treatment of osteoporosis. Numerous double-blind placebo-controlled trials have shown that treatment with alendronate and risedronate decreases the risks of vertebral and hip fractures by 50%. Ibandronate has been shown to decrease the risk of vertebral fractures, but the data is not compelling regarding a decrease in the risk of hip fractures. Bisphosphonates may offer lesser value in the setting of untreated vitamin D deficiency.

The intravenous preparations are often used when compliance or GI tolerability may be a concern. **Table 15.7** outlines the available bisphosphonate options for the treatment of osteoporosis. Once the decision is made to use one of these drugs, the patient must be informed to take calcium as well as vitamin D supplements in the doses outlined earlier. Tolerability, adverse events, and duration of therapy are at times limiting factors in the utilization of this drug class. The oral absorption of these drugs is very poor, hence they must be taken on an empty stomach with at least 8 ounces of tap water and then the patient must remain upright for 45 minutes to an hour and not take anything else orally during this time frame. Oral preparations may cause nausea and esophagitis, which can be severe. Other adverse side effects include arthralgias and myalgias (both of which can rarely be severe and last for weeks to months), hypocalcaemia, gastric as well as esophageal ulcerations, and rarely uveitis (questionable association). The most serious adverse event that has been associated with the bisphosphonates is osteonecrosis of the jaw (ONJ) and a questionable link with the development of esophageal cancer.[6] Prior to starting therapy, patients may be advised to make sure that any anticipated dental work has been completed (particularly a tooth extraction), and, if required during administration, cessation of these agents for 2 to 3 months may at times be recommended before having dental work. The incidence of ONJ is rare even in the highest risk group, being those treated with the intravenous preparations for neoplastic disease (when the dose administered is commonly 12 times that used for treatment of osteoporosis). Intravenous preparations are to be avoided in renal insufficiency (creatinine clearance <30 mg/mL). Although there have been case reports of these medications being safe during pregnancy, current recommendations are to avoid these agents in pregnancy and in women of child-bearing age, because these agents essentially are bound to bone for years and are not entirely excreted.

Table 15.7 Currently Available Bisphosphonate Therapies

Formulation	Dose Options
Oral	
Alendronate	10 mg daily or 70 mg weekly
Risedronate	5 mg daily or 35 mg weekly
Ibandronate	2.5 mg daily or 150 mg monthly
Etidronate	400 mg daily for 2 weeks, every 3 months

(continues)

Table 15.7   Currently Available Bisphosphonate Therapies, cont'd

FORMULATION	DOSE OPTIONS
Parenteral	
Ibandronate	3 mg IV, every 3 months
Zoledronic acid	5 mg IV, yearly

The two intravenous preparations that are available for use include zoledronic acid and ibandronate. Both are very effective therapies, but zoledronic acid has better outcome data in showing a decrease in hip and vertebral fractures, can be given once yearly, and a recent study showed that it can improve morbidity and mortality if given within 3 months of a hip fracture.[7] Adverse events of intravenous therapies (other than GI tolerance) are similar to those for oral preparations. They have also been associated with headaches and rarely nephrotic syndrome. The evidence is conflicting regarding atrial fibrillation as an adverse event secondary to zoledronic acid therapy.

Once the decision is made to treat with this class of drugs, one must decide on the duration. One can use bone mineral density measurements to help determine treatment, but fracture risk improves even in the absence of dramatic improvements in bone density. Although it is unclear exactly how long patients should be treated, studies have shown that fracture prevention after 5 years of therapy may persist for 5 more years after cessation of therapy.[8] The proper duration of bisphophonate therapy remains an open question as outlined in a recent secondary analysis and accompanying discussion.[9,10]

Estrogen Replacement Therapy and Selective Estrogen Receptor Modulators

Without question, estrogen replacement therapy (ERT) is effective in the treatment of osteoporosis. Multiple studies have shown that ERT may decrease the rates of hip and vertebral fractures by 25% and 50%, respectively. However, as long-term experience has accumulated with these agents, the risk profile has shifted. These agents appear to increase the risk of breast cancer, stroke, heart disease, uterine cancer, thromboembolic disease, mood disorders, and gallbladder disease. For these reasons, these agents are no longer the first-line therapy for treatment of osteoporosis. Certainly, they are very effective in symptomatic treatment of menopausal symptoms. It may also be advisable to use these agents in premature menopause or for symptomatic relief of menopausal symptoms for a more limited interval and then transition to other agents to treat osteoporosis. When using estrogens, progestin analogues should be administered to patients who have not had a hysterectomy to protect the uterine lining.

Raloxifine, a selective estrogen receptor modulator (SERM), has been approved by the FDA for the treatment and prevention of osteoporosis. This agent decreases the risk of vertebral fractures, but it has not been shown to decrease the risk of nonvertebral fractures. It may actually decrease the risk of breast cancer and heart disease and stroke in those patients who are at higher risk profiles. However, the drug may exacerbate menopausal symptoms and retain the risk of thromboembolic disease and is thus not an option for the treatment of menopausal symptoms.

Teriparatide

Teriparatide is a parathyroid hormone analogue and is the only anabolic agent that has been approved by the FDA for the treatment of osteoporosis. It has been shown to decrease vertebral and nonvertebral fractures and, when compared to alendronate, it decreased fractures to a greater extent. The drug is administered subcutaneously daily. It should not be administered for longer than 18 to 24 months. In addition, if it is used after therapy with a bisphosphonate, the clinical effectiveness may be blunted and a delay of 3 or more months after bisphosphonate use is often advised before initiating teriparitide. Although it appears to be the most effective agent and the only truly anabolic agent available to treat osteoporosis, it carries a "black box" warning due to the development of osteosarcomas in laboratory rats that had been administered relatively large doses in animal studies. Due to this warning, the drug is relatively contraindicated in patients who have had skeletal irradiation, Paget's disease, a history of cancers of the bone or those that may metastasize to bone, as well as those patients who have hypercalcemia (a relatively common transient adverse event from the drug) or who are pregnant or nursing. Due to these safety issues and lack of longer-term clinical experience, this agent is currently reserved for those patients with severe osteoporosis or who have failed, cannot tolerate, or are inappropriate candidates for the other listed therapies. While enhanced bone density induced by bisphosphonates tends to remain for at least several years after their discontinuation, there is a rapid decline in bone density after discontinuation of teriparatide. Initiation of a bisphosphonate is therefore generally advised immediately upon discontinuation of teriparatide after completion of its usual two year course.

Calcitonin

Calcitonin has been shown to relieve bone pain from acute compression fractures but with inconsistent observed benefit. It has also been shown to decrease vertebral fractures, but not hip fractures. It is administered either subcutaneously or as a nasal spray. Adverse reactions are uncommon, but it is felt that its clinical effects are not as potent as the other agents outlined and its long term use clinically has been difficult to maintain.

Future Directions

Denosumab is a biologic therapy in development for the treatment of osteoporosis. It is a humanized monoclonal antibody that will be administered subcutaneously every 6 months. It blocks the RANK-ligand, thus decreasing osteoclast activation. There is enthusiasm that this agent may be yet another effective alternative for the treatment of postmenopausal osteoporosis. At the same time, there is concern that as an immune modulator, there may be risk associated with response to infection or that its use may promote tumor development or progression.

STEROID-INDUCED OSTEOPOROSIS

Glucocorticoid therapy is widely used for a multitude of medical problems. Their use is so widespread that some studies in the United Kingdom have estimated that at any one time up to 1% of the entire population is using a steroid medication, and for those patients aged 70 to 79 years, the estimate of use increases to 2.4%. The long-term adverse events associated with steroids are well known, but in particular include skin fragility, diabetes, weight gain, hypertension, and osteoporosis, among others. Unfortunately there is no "safe" long-term dose of steroids, because bone loss has been correlated with inhaled steroids and oral doses as low as 2.5 mg/day of prednisone equivalent. In addition, it is well known that bone is lost rapidly with the initiation of steroid use, increasing fracture risk, and both bone loss and risk of fracture fall when steroids are stopped. In addition, patients on steroids may experience fragility fractures out of proportion to their bone density level. The evaluation and initial treatment of patients for osteoporosis who are on steroids includes bone density measurements; appropriate calcium and vitamin D supplementation; exercise; and avoidance of other risk factors for bone loss, as well as attention to the other parameters previously outlined. It appears that use of the bisphosphonates risedronate, alendronate, etidronate, as well as zoledronic acid as treatment for steroid-induced osteoporosis has decreased the risk of vertebral fractures. The FDA has approved the use of risedronate, alendronate, and zoledronic acid for treatment of postmenopausal osteoporosis. Teriparatide has been shown to increase bone mass in patients with steroid induced osteoporosis.

The American College of Rheumatology's recommendations for the prevention and treatment of glucocorticoid-induced osteoporosis are summarized in **Table 15.8**.

Table 15.8   Recommendations for the Prevention and Treatment of Glucocorticoid-Induced Osteoporosis[11]

Patients initiating therapy at 5 mg/day prednisone equivalent or greater and planned duration for >3 months:
- Modify lifestyle risk factors for osteoporosis:
- Smoking cessation
- Reduction of alcohol consumption
- Weight-bearing exercise
- Calcium supplementation
- Vitamin D supplementation
- Initiate bisphosphonate therapy (caution in women of childbearing age)

(continues)

Table 15.8 Recommendations for the Prevention and Treatment of Glucocorticoid-Induced Osteoporosis,[11] cont'd

Patients receiving long-term therapy at dose of prednisone 5 mg/day or equivalent
- Modify lifestyle risk factors for osteoporosis:
- Smoking cessation
- Reduction of alcohol consumption
- Weight-bearing exercise
- Calcium supplementation
- Vitamin D supplementation
- Consider hormone replacement therapy if deficient or clinically indicated (controversial)

Measure bone mineral density: T score below −1.0
- Prescribe bisphosphonate (caution in women of childbearing age)
- Consider alternative pharmacologic agent if contraindication of unable to tolerate bisphosphonate therapy
- Repeat bone mineral density test annually or biannually.

REFERENCES

1. Burge R, Dawson-Hughes B, Solomon DH, Wong JB, King A, Tosteson A. Incidence and economic burden of osteoporosis-related fractures in the United States, 2005–2025. *J Bone Miner Res.* 2007;22:365–475.

2. Clinician's Guide to Prevention and Treatment of Osteoporosis. Washington, DC: National Osteoporosis Foundation; 2010. Available online at www.nof.org.

3. Qaseem A, Snow V, Shekelle P, et al. Screening for osteoporosis in men: a clinical practice guideline from the American College of Physicians. *Ann Intern Med.* 2008;148:680–684.

4. Lewiecki A, Watts N. New guidelines for the treatment of osteoporosis. *South Med J.* 2009;102:175–179.

5. National Osteoporosis Foundation. Osteoporosis Clinical Update: Update on Bisphosphonates FDA-approved for Prevention and Treatment of Osteoporosis. July 2008. Available online at www.nof.org.

6. Khosla S. Bisphosphonate-associated osteonecrosis of the jaw: Report of a task force of the American Society for Bone and Mineral Research. *J Bone Miner Res.* 2007;22(10):1470–1489.

7. Lyles KW, Colón-Emeric CS, Magaziner JS, et al. Zoledronic acid and clinical fractures and mortality after hip fracture. *N Engl J Med.* 2007;357:1799–1809.

8. Black DM, Schwartz AV, Ensrud KE, et al. Effects of continuing or stopping alendronate after 5 years of treatment. The Fracture Intervention Trial Long Term Extension (FLEX): A randomized trial. *JAMA.* 2006;296(24):2927–2938.

9. Black DM, Kelly MP, Genant HK, et al. Bisphosphonates and fractures of the subtrochanteric or diaphyseal femur. *N Engl J Med.* 2010 Mar 24. [Epub ahead of print]

10. Shane E. Evolving data about subtrochanteric fractures and bisphosphonates. *N Engl J Med.* 2010 Mar 24. [Epub ahead of print]

11. Buckley L and the ACR Ad Hoc Committee on Glucocorticoid-Induced Osteoporosis. Recommendations for the prevention and treatment of glucocorticoid-induced osteoporosis. *Arth Rheum.* 2001:44(7):1496–1503.

◇◇◇◇◇◇◇◇◇◇◇◇◇◇◇◇◇◇◇◇◇◇◇◇

SUGGESTED READINGS

Bone and Tooth Society of Great Britain. National Osteoporosis Society. Royal College of Physicians. Royal College of Physicians of London. *Glucocorticoid-induced Osteoporosis: Guidelines for Prevention and Treatment.* Sudbury, Suffolk (Britain): Lavenham Press; 2002.

Bringhurst FR, Demay MB, Krane SM, Kronenberg HM. Bone and mineral metabolism in health and disease. In: Kasper DL, Braunwald E, Fauci AS, et al, eds. *Harrison's Principles of Internal Medicine*, 16th ed. New York: McGraw-Hill, 2005:2238–2249.

Fuvus MJ (ed). *Primer on the Metabolic Bone Diseases and Disorders of Mineral Metabolism,* 6th ed. Washington, DC: American Society of Bone and Mineral Research; 2006.

Hakim A, Clunie G, Haq I. *Oxford Handbook of Rheumatology*, 2nd ed. New York: Oxford University Press; 2006.

Klippel JH. *Primer on the Rheumatic Diseases,* 12th ed. Atlanta, GA: Arthritis Foundation; 2001.

Miller PD, Leonard MB. Radiological evaluation of bone mineral in children. In: Fuvus MJ (ed)., *Primer on the Metabolic Bone Diseases and Disorders of Mineral Metabolism,* 6th ed. Washington, DC: American Society of Bone and Mineral Research; 2006.

Nelson HD, et al. Screening for postmenopausal osteoporosis: a review of the evidence for the U.S. Preventive Task Force. *Ann Intern Med.* 2002;137: 529.

U.S. Preventive Services Task Force (USPSTF). Screening for Osteoporosis in Postmenopausal Women: Recommendations and Rationale. Rockville, MD: Agency for Healthcare Research and Quality (AHRQ); 2002.

CHAPTER 16

Overview of Pharmacologic Therapy in the Rheumatic Diseases: Indications and Risks

Sonali Desai, MD

OVERVIEW

A multitude of medications are available for the treatment of rheumatic diseases. These therapeutics include non-steroidal anti-inflammatory drugs (NSAIDs), disease-modifying antirheumatic drugs (DMARDs), systemic glucocorticoids, immunosuppressives, and biologic agents. Each therapy must be chosen carefully in order to balance the potential benefits of the medication with its associated toxicities. A detailed review of all pharmacologic options for each rheumatic disease is beyond the scope of this chapter; however, a general overview of the approach to drug therapy in the rheumatic diseases is provided, with a focus on the most prevalent condition, rheumatoid arthritis (RA).

NONSTEROIDAL ANTI-INFLAMMATORY DRUGS

NSAIDs represent one of the most frequently used classes of medications and are not specific to rheumatology. NSAIDs alleviate pain and reduce inflammation; two of the cardinal features of arthritis, and they are often used to treat osteoarthritis. NSAIDs are also used as a first-line approach for musculoskeletal pain, including arthralgias and arthritis. They are not true disease-modifying therapies or immunosuppressives; they may not halt the progression of rheumatic disease, but they can be effective in the treatment of its symptoms. NSAIDs do carry several key side effects, including gastrointestinal, renal, and cardiovascular risks, which must be thoughtfully assessed in the individual patient treated with this class of medications. Patients at risk for gastrointestinal bleeding should be treated concomitantly with either misoprostol or a proton-pump inhibitor.[1] Other less common but potentially harmful effects are allergic reactions; hepatotoxicity; and pulmonary, hematologic, and central nervous system problems. **Table 16.1** reviews some of the more commonly prescribed NSAIDs and their dosages.

Table 16.1   NSAIDs Commonly Used in the Treatment of Arthralgias and Arthritis

NSAID	DOSAGE
Aspirin	2.4–5.4 g per day
Ibuprofen	200–800 mg up to four times per day
Naproxen	225–500 mg twice daily
Indomethacin	25–50 mg up to four times per day
Diclofenac	50–75 mg twice daily
Etodolac	200–300 mg twice to four times per day
Piroxicam	10–20 mg per day
Nabumetone	500 mg twice daily
Celecoxib	100–200 mg twice per day

CORTICOSTEROIDS

Corticosteroids represent a double-edged sword in the treatment of rheumatic diseases. They are highly efficacious in the short-term treatment of many inflammatory conditions, such as systemic vasculidites and flares of systemic lupus erythematosus (SLE) and RA. However, their adverse effects are just as potent and often preclude their long-term use. The toxicities of corticosteroids have been well studied and include, but are not limited to, osteoporosis, hypertension, weight gain, hyperglycemia, alterations in mood, increased susceptibility to infections, and cataracts.[2]

Generally, corticosteroids are used to treat acute flares of rheumatic disease, severe systemic inflammation, or as a bridge therapy in diseases such as RA. Once disease remission is achieved, steroid-sparing agents are often introduced and corticosteroids are tapered in order to maximize therapeutic effects and minimize known adverse effects. Vigilance for the development of adrenal insufficiency is essential during this tapering period, because corticosteroids suppress the endogenous hypothalamic–pituitary axis. Because of the risk of osteoporosis, patients on steroids should receive calcium and vitamin D; antiresorptive therapy should also be considered. **Table 16.2** provides an overview of the average dose of corticosteroids used to treat different rheumatic diseases.

Table 16.2   Corticosteroid Dosages Used to Treat Different Rheumatic Diseases

DISEASE	CORTICOSTEROID	DOSE
Severe organ-threatening disease flare (RA, SLE, systemic vasculitis)	Methylprednisolone	250–1000 mg per day for 3 days
Giant cell arteritis	Prednisone	60 mg per day
Inflammatory myopathy (dermatomyositis, polymyositis)	Prednisone	1 mg/kg per day
Polymyalgia rheumatica	Prednisone	15–20 mg per day
RA flare or bridge therapy or SLE flare	Prednisone	10–30 mg per day

DISEASE-MODIFYING ANTIRHEUMATIC DRUGS

Table 16.3 lists some of the currently available DMARDs used in the treatment of rheumatic diseases.

Table 16.3   Dosing of DMARD and Immunosuppressive Therapies in Rheumatic Diseases

MEDICATION	ADMINISTRATION ROUTE	DOSE
Hydroxychloroquine	Oral	6.5 mg/kg per day (average dose 200 mg twice daily)
Sulfasalazine	Oral	Starting dose 500 mg per day Goal 3000 mg per day
Methotrexate	Oral or subcutaneous	Starting dose 7.5–10 mg per week Maximal dose 25 mg per week
Leflunomide	Oral	10–20 mg per day
Azathioprine	Oral	Starting dose 50 mg per day Goal 2.0–2.5 mg/kg
Mycophenolate mofetil	Oral	Starting dose 500 mg per day Goal 3000 mg per day (1500 mg twice daily)
Cyclophosphamide	Oral or IV	2 mg/kg/day orally Starting 750–1000 mg/m^2 IV Subsequent 500–1000 mg/m^2 IV (based on nadir white blood cell count and patient response)

Hydroxychloroquine and Chloroquine

Hydroxychloroquine and chloroquine are antimalarial compounds that are used to treat mild RA and SLE either as monotherapy or in combination with other DMARDs.[3,4] They are generally well tolerated, with gastrointestinal side effects being the most common. Retinal toxicity is rare; however, routine annual ophthalmologic screening is recommended. The dosing of hydroxychloroquine is ideally maintained at doses of less than 6.5 mg/kg, because the toxicity of this medication is dose-related. The most frequently used dosing regimen is 200 mg twice daily. It can take from 12 to 24 weeks for hydroxychloroquine to demonstrate a positive therapeutic effect.

Sulfasalazine

Sulfasalazine is a combination of sulfapyridine and 5-aminosalicylic acid used in the treatment of RA, psoriatic arthritis, and the peripheral arthritis of ankylosing spondylitis. Its primary side effects are gastrointestinal, with nausea and abdominal discomfort occurring frequently.[5] Other known toxicities include leukopenia, a decrease in sperm counts in males, and central nervous system effects.[6] One unique adverse effect is a syndrome of fever, rash, and elevated liver function tests; if this condition occurs, the patient must stop the medication immediately.[7]

Sulfasalazine is generally started at a low dose with gradual uptitration and close laboratory monitoring (complete blood count, liver function tests).[8] The starting dose is 500 mg/day with a maximum dose of 3000 mg/day, depending on how well the medication is tolerated and how efficacious it is for the individual patient. It can take up to 12 weeks for the benefits of therapy with sulfasalazine to become manifest. Close monitoring of the complete blood count (CBC) is required in the initial several months of starting this drug, because neutropenia tends to occur early in the course of therapy.

Methotrexate

Methotrexate is a cornerstone of DMARD therapy in the management of RA.[9,10] It is also used in a variety of other rheumatic conditions, such as psoriatic arthritis, inflammatory myopathies, and SLE. Methotrexate is taken once per week either orally or subcutaneously with a starting dose of 7.5 to 10 mg per week and a maximal dose in inflammatory arthritis of 25 mg per week (higher doses are often used in inflammatory myopathies). Daily folic acid or weekly folinic acid (leucovorin) supplementation is concomitantly prescribed to ameliorate many of the side effects. It is generally well tolerated, and routine bloodwork is required (CBC, liver function tests, renal function) more frequently when the medication is first started or major dose changes occur and then every 8 to 12 weeks for ongoing therapy.[11] Patients who have chronic liver disease; alcohol abuse; significant renal impairment; chronic infections, including hepatitis B or C; and those with significant lung disease should not receive methotrexate. Patients may not experience a decrease in their arthritis until at least 4 weeks after starting therapeutic doses of methotrexate.

The more common side effects of methotrexate include gastrointestinal toxicity, stomatitis, and fatigue. The most serious adverse effects of methotrexate also include lung injury, liver toxicity, cytopenias, and a rare risk of lymphoma. Methotrexate is cleared by the kidneys; thus, its dose must be modified based on the glomerular filtration rate and it should not be used in patients who have renal failure or are on dialysis. The intake of significant quantities of alcohol is not recommended in patients taking methotrexate due to the potential hepatotoxic effect. Patients should also be screened for hepatitis B and C and if positive, alternative therapies, including concomitant antiviral therapies, should be considered. In addition, methotrexate is a known teratogen; and women of childbearing age should not use it.[12] Because trimethoprim-sulfamethoxazole is a potent antifolate therapy when combined with methotrexate, there is an increase risk of bone marrow toxicity, so this combination should be avoided.[13]

Leflunomide

Leflunomide is primarily used for RA, often in patients who have failed methotrexate, cannot tolerate methotrexate, or in combination with methotrexate or other DMARDs. It is given at a dose of 10 to 20 mg per day and is similar in efficacy to methotrexate.[14] The most common side effect is diarrhea, but other adverse reactions include rash, alopecia, cytopenias, and liver function test abnormalities. Routine lab monitoring is recommended (CBC and liver function tests). Interstitial lung disease has been reported, but its true association with leflunomide is somewhat controversial.[15] Leflunomide should not be taken by women of childbearing age who are pregnant or who plan to become pregnant.

Azathioprine

Azathioprine is primarily used as a corticosteroid-sparing agent in the management of SLE, inflammatory myopathy, and vasculitis; it can be used to treat RA, but it is generally not an effective first-line agent in RA.[16] The usual dosing of azathioprine is a starting regimen of 25 to 50 mg per day with an increase to 2 to 2.5 mg/kg in a few weeks. The primary side effects associated with azathioprine include leucopenia and gastrointestinal symptoms. Hypersensitivity reactions can occur rarely and lead to discontinuation of the medication. Genetic testing of thiopurine methyltransferase (TMPT) enzyme activity may correlate with an increased risk of the development of toxicity and is often performed prior to initiating therapy with azathioprine; however, patients with normal enzyme activity may still develop toxicity.[17,18] Close lab monitoring for leukopenia with complete blood counts is required with azathioprine. One dangerous drug interaction with azathioprine is worth noting: allopurinol, a medication used in the chronic management of gout, can lead to an increase in the toxicity of azathioprine. The concomitant administration of these two medications necessitates a dose-reduction of azathioprine and close clinical monitoring of the patient to prevent toxicity.

IMMUNOSUPPRESSIVE MEDICATIONS

Mycophenolate Mofetil

Mycophenolate mofetil is primarily used in the treatment of SLE nephritis, but also plays a role as a corticosteroid-sparing agent in inflammatory myopathy and vasculitis.[19] The doses utilized in the treatment of rheumatic diseases start at 500 mg per day, with the ultimate goal of 1500 to 3000 mg per day, in divided doses. The main adverse effects noted with this medication are gastrointestinal problems (nausea, diarrhea, and abdominal discomfort) and cytopenias.[20] Viral infections such as herpes zoster and cytomegalovirus have been reported in patients taking this medication.[21,22] Mycophenolate mofetil is contraindicated in women of childbearing age who are pregnant or who are considering pregnancy. Lab monitoring with CBCs should be performed more frequently at the initiation of this drug and then routinely thereafter.

Cyclophosphamide

Cyclophosphamide is an immunosuppressive agent used for several of the more severe manifestations of rheumatic disease, including renal and neurologic complications of SLE; Wegener's granulomatosis, as well as other vasculidites; and rheumatic disease-associated interstitial lung disease. The medication is given either through the intravenous or oral route, depending on the indication. Routine complete blood count with differential monitoring is performed every 1 to 2 weeks during both oral and intravenous administration. The dosing for oral cyclophosphamide is generally 2 mg/kg per day, with adjustment for impaired renal function. The dosing for intravenous cyclophosphamide is 750 to 1000 mg/m^2 initially, followed by 500 to 1000 mg/m^2, depending on the nadir white blood cell count and patient response to the first dose. Dose-related leukopenia is common, but if the total white blood cell count is <3500/mm^3, then the dose of cyclophosphamide should be decreased.

Cyclophosphamide is efficacious, but this high-potency drug also carries several important risks. Hemmorhagic cystitis and bladder cancer have been well described.[23] Hematologic malignancies may also occur years after cyclophosphamide exposure. Toxicity to the reproductive organs, ovarian failure in women and azoospermia in men, is a chief concern for younger patients. These important concerns must be addressed with the patient before considering the administration of this toxic therapy.

ANTI-TUMOR NECROSIS FACTOR-THERAPIES

The tumor necrosis factor-α (TNF-α) inhibitors include infliximab, etanercept, adalimumab, certolizumab, and golimumab. These agents have had a substantial impact on the treatment of RA, psoriatic arthritis, and ankylosing spondylitis, both in terms of their ability to reduce joint pain and inflammation and their effect on radiographic progression. The TNF-α inhibitors are efficacious as monotherapy, but all have increased effectiveness when used with methotrexate for the treatment of RA.[24–31]

These therapies are generally used for moderate-to-severe joint disease in RA. Practice patterns on the timing of biologic therapies for RA vary in different parts of the world, but in the United States they are generally reserved for patients who fail therapy with DMARDs, primarily methotrexate, or who are not candidates for DMARDs. In ankylosing spondylitis and psoriatic arthritis, patients who have active disease or have failed other therapies can be treated with TNF-α inhibitors.[32]

The definitive adverse effects of the TNF-α inhibitors include administration reactions (injection site with etanercept and adalimumab; infusion reactions with infliximab), drug-induced lupus demyelinating syndromes, and increased infection risk. The immunosuppressive effect of these agents results in a higher risk of many serious infections, such as bacterial infections, and opportunistic infections, including fungal disease and mycobacterial infections. Reactivation of latent tuberculosis (TB) has been reported and may be higher with infliximab compared to etanercept.[33,34] Patients screened for TB with a purified protein derivative (PPD) skin test prior to starting therapy and those with evidence of latent TB should receive appropriate antimicrobial therapies. Additionally, the pneumococcal vaccine, as well as annual flu vaccines, are recommended prior to starting biologics. Several other concerns with TNF-α inhibitors have arisen in the post-marketing period, including heart failure, cytopenias, and hepatotoxicity. A putative increase in the risk of malignancy has also been reported (lymphoma, solid organ, and skin); however, this has not been conclusively proven, except for non melanoma skin cancers.

OTHER BIOLOGIC THERAPIES

B cell depletion (rituximab), costimulation blockade (abatacept), and interleukin 6 (IL-6) receptor antagonism (tocilizumab) are three other therapeutic approaches that have been developed to treat RA.[35-42] Rituximab and tocilizumab are generally reserved for patients who have failed or who are not candidates for TNF-α inhibitors, whereas abatacept may be used in patients who have not responded to other DMARDs but who are TNF-α inhibitors naive. As with all of these therapies, the risk of infection may be increased. Patients who have chronic hepatitis B infection should not receive anti-TNF or the other biologics. A summary of the dosing for TNF-α inhibitors and biologic agents is provided in **Table 16.4**.

Table 16.4   Dosing of the TNF-α Inhibitors and Biologic Therapies for Rheumatoid Arthritis

THERAPY	ROUTE	DOSE
Infliximab	Intravenous	3 mg/kg at 0, 2, 6 weeks, then 3 to 10 mg/kg every 4 to 8 weeks
Etanercept	Subcutaneous	50 mg once weekly or 25 mg twice weekly
Adalimumab	Subcutaneous	40 mg every other week 40 mg every week (if not taking concomitant methotrexate)
Golimumab	Subcutaneous	50 mg once monthly
Certolizumab	Subcutaneous	400 mg first dose 400 mg at week 2 and week 4 Maintenance: 200 mg every other week or 400 mg once monthly
Rituximab	Intravenous	1000 mg on day 1 1000 mg on day 15 Recommendations for subsequent dosing based on clinical judgment
Abatacept	Intravenous	Dosing is weight-based at 1, 2, and 4 weeks Repeat dose every 4 weeks thereafter <60 kg = 500 mg 60–100 kg = 750 mg >100 kg = 1000 mg
Tocilizumab	Intravenous	4 mg/kg starting dose 8 mg/kg based on clinical response

MONITORING DRUG THERAPY

In order to mitigate the possible side effects associated with the treatment of rheumatic diseases, frequent monitoring is often needed. In RA, for example, specific guidelines have been put forth to screen for toxicity.[11,43] A summary of these guidelines and the recommendations in this chapter are provided as a framework for following patients on rheumatic disease therapy (**Table 16.5**).

Table 16.5   Suggested Monitoring Guidelines for RA Drug Therapy

MEDICATION	MONITORING
NSAIDs	CBC, BUN/Cr
Glucocorticoids	Eye exam, blood pressure, bone density, serum glucose, fasting lipids
Hydroxychloroquine	Eye exam (fundoscopic, visual fields)
Sulfasalazine	CBC, LFTs
Methotrexate	Hepatitis B and C testing at baseline CBC, LFTs, albumin, BUN/Cr
Leflunomide	CBC, LFTs, BUN/Cr
Azathioprine	CBC, LFTs
Mycophenolate mofetil	CBC, LFTs
Cyclophosphamide	CBC, urinalysis
Biologic therapies (infliximab, etanercept, adalimumab, golimumab, certolizumab, rituximab, abatacept)	Pre-initiation: immunization status, PPD, hepatitis B and C testing at baseline Ongoing therapy: complete CBC

CBC = complete blood count, LFTs = liver function tests, BUN/Cr = renal function, PPD = purified protein derivative.

SUMMARY

In summary, there are a variety of medications available to treat the rheumatic diseases, with many more in the early phases of drug development. Balancing the risks of medication toxicities with their therapeutic benefits and monitoring the side effects of therapy closely is essential to achieving a good clinical response. The focus of this chapter has been on the treatment options for rheumatoid arthritis, but many of the principles of treatment apply to other rheumatic diseases with dose and duration adjustments.

◇◇◇◇◇◇◇◇◇◇◇◇

REFERENCES

1. Recommendations for use of selective and nonselective nonsteroidal antiinflammatory drugs: an American College of Rheumatology white paper. *Arthritis Rheum.* 2008;59(8):1058–1073.

2. McDonough AK, Curtis JR, Saag KG. The epidemiology of glucocorticoid-associated adverse events. *Curr Opin Rheumatol.* 2008;20(2):131–137.

3. Clark P, Casas E, Tugwell P, et al. Hydroxychloroquine compared with placebo in rheumatoid arthritis. A randomized controlled trial. *Ann Intern Med.* 1993;119(11):1067–1071.

4. Ruiz-Irastorza G, Ramos-Casals M, Brito-Zeron P, Khamashta MA. Clinical efficacy and side effects of antimalarials in systemic lupus erythematosus: a systematic review. *Ann Rheum Dis.* 2010;69(1):20–28

5. Donahue KE, Gartlehner G, Jonas DE, et al. Systematic review: comparative effectiveness and harms of disease-modifying medications for rheumatoid arthritis. *Ann Intern Med.* 2008;148(2):124–134.

6. Farr M, Scott DG, Bacon PA. Side effect profile of 200 patients with inflammatory arthritides treated with sulphasalazine. *Drugs.* 1986;32(Suppl 1):49–53.

7. Fuchs HA. Use of sulfasalazine in rheumatic diseases. *Bull Rheum Dis.* 1997;46(7):3–4.

8. van Riel PL, van Gestel AM, van de Putte LB. Long-term usage and side-effect profile of sulphasalazine in rheumatoid arthritis. *Br J Rheumatol.* 1995;34(Suppl 2):40–42.

9. Weinblatt ME, Coblyn JS, Fox DA, et al. Efficacy of low-dose methotrexate in rheumatoid arthritis. *N Engl J Med.* 1985;312(13):818–822.

10. Andersen PA, West SG, O'Dell JR, Via CS, Claypool RG, Kotzin BL. Weekly pulse methotrexate in rheumatoid arthritis. Clinical and immunologic effects in a randomized, double-blind study. *Ann Intern Med.* Oct 1985;103(4):489–496.

11. Saag KG, Teng GG, Patkar NM, et al. American College of Rheumatology 2008 recommendations for the use of nonbiologic and biologic disease-modifying antirheumatic drugs in rheumatoid arthritis. *Arthritis Rheum.* 2008;59(6):762–784.

12. Buckley LM, Bullaboy CA, Leichtman L, Marquez M. Multiple congenital anomalies associated with weekly low-dose methotrexate treatment of the mother. *Arthritis Rheum.* May 1997;40(5):971–973.

13. Jones KW, Patel SR. A family physician's guide to monitoring methotrexate. *Am Fam Physician.* 2000;62(7):1607–1612, 1614.

14. Cohen SB, Iqbal I. Leflunomide. *Int J Clin Pract.* 2003;57(2):115–120.

15. Suissa S, Hudson M, Ernst P. Leflunomide use and the risk of interstitial lung disease in rheumatoid arthritis. *Arthritis Rheum.* 2006;54(5):1435–1439.

16. Willkens RF, Urowitz MB, Stablein DM, et al. Comparison of azathioprine, methotrexate, and the combination of both in the treatment of rheumatoid arthritis. A controlled clinical trial. *Arthritis Rheum.* 1992;35(8):849–856.

17. Clunie GP, Lennard L. Relevance of thiopurine methyltransferase status in rheumatology patients receiving azathioprine. *Rheumatology (Oxford).* 2004;43(1):13–18.

18. Sanderson J, Ansari A, Marinaki T, Duley J. Thiopurine methyltransferase: should it be measured before commencing thiopurine drug therapy? *Ann Clin Biochem.* 2004;41(Pt 4):294–302.

19. Contreras G, Sosnov J. Role of mycophenolate mofetil in the treatment of lupus nephritis. *Clin J Am Soc Nephrol.* 2007;2(5):879–882.

20. Riskalla MM, Somers EC, Fatica RA, McCune WJ. Tolerability of mycophenolate mofetil in patients with systemic lupus erythematosus. *J Rheumatol.* 2003;30(7):1508–1512.

21. Buell C, Koo J. Long-term safety of mycophenolate mofetil and cyclosporine: a review. *J Drugs Dermatol.* 2008;7(8):741–748.

22. F L, Y T, X P, et al. A prospective multicentre study of mycophenolate mofetil combined with prednisolone as induction therapy in 213 patients with active lupus nephritis. *Lupus.* 2008;17(7):622–629.

23. Talar-Williams C, Hijazi YM, Walther MM, et al. Cyclophosphamide-induced cystitis and bladder cancer in patients with Wegener granulomatosis. *Ann Intern Med.* 1996;124(5):477–484.

24. Weinblatt ME, Keystone EC, Furst DE, et al. Adalimumab, a fully human anti-tumor necrosis factor alpha monoclonal antibody, for the treatment of rheumatoid arthritis in patients taking concomitant methotrexate: the ARMADA trial. *Arthritis Rheum.* 2003;48(1):35–45.

25. Maini RN, Breedveld FC, Kalden JR, et al. Therapeutic efficacy of multiple intravenous infusions of anti-tumor necrosis factor alpha monoclonal antibody combined with low-dose weekly methotrexate in rheumatoid arthritis. *Arthritis Rheum.* 1998;41(9):1552–1563.

26. Klareskog L, van der Heijde D, de Jager JP, et al. Therapeutic effect of the combination of etanercept and methotrexate compared with each treatment alone in patients with rheumatoid arthritis: double-blind randomised controlled trial. *Lancet.* 2004;363(9410):675–681.

27. Emery P, Fleischmann RM, Moreland LW, et al. Golimumab, a human anti-tumor necrosis factor alpha monoclonal antibody, injected subcutaneously every four weeks in methotrexate-naive patients with active rheumatoid arthritis: twenty-four-week results of a phase III, multicenter, randomized, double-blind, placebo-controlled study of golimumab before methotrexate as first-line therapy for early-onset rheumatoid arthritis. *Arthritis Rheum.* 2009;60(8):2272–2283.

28. Keystone EC, Genovese MC, Klareskog L, et al. Golimumab, a human antibody to tumour necrosis factor {alpha} given by monthly subcutaneous injections, in active rheumatoid arthritis despite methotrexate therapy: the GO-FORWARD Study. *Ann Rheum Dis.* 2009;68(6):789–796.

29. Smolen J, Landewé RB, Mease P, et al. Efficacy and safety of certolizumab pegol plus methotrexate in active rheumatoid arthritis: the RAPID 2 study. A randomised controlled trial. *Ann Rheum Dis.* 2009;68(6):797–804.

30. Fleischmann R, Vencovsky J, van Vollenhoven RF, et al. Efficacy and safety of certolizumab pegol monotherapy every 4 weeks in patients with rheumatoid arthritis failing previous disease-modifying antirheumatic therapy: the FAST4WARD study. *Ann Rheum Dis.* 2009;68(6):805–811.

31. Kay J, Matteson EL, Dasgupta B, et al. Golimumab in patients with active rheumatoid arthritis despite treatment with methotrexate: a randomized, double-blind, placebo-controlled, dose-ranging study. *Arthritis Rheum.* 2008;58(4):964–975.

32. Braun J, Davis J, Dougados M, Sieper J, van der Linden S, van der Heijde D. First update of the international ASAS consensus statement for the use of anti-TNF agents in patients with ankylosing spondylitis. *Ann Rheum Dis.* 2006;65(3):316–320.

33. Gomez-Reino JJ, Carmona L, Valverde VR, Mola EM, Montero MD. Treatment of rheumatoid arthritis with tumor necrosis factor inhibitors may predispose to significant increase in tuberculosis risk: a multicenter active-surveillance report. *Arthritis Rheum.* 2003;48(8):2122–2127.

34. Askling J, Fored CM, Brandt L, et al. Risk and case characteristics of tuberculosis in rheumatoid arthritis associated with tumor necrosis factor antagonists in Sweden. *Arthritis Rheum.* 2005;52(7):1986–1992.

35. Cohen SB, Emery P, Greenwald MW, et al. Rituximab for rheumatoid arthritis refractory to anti-tumor necrosis factor therapy: Results of a multicenter, randomized, double-blind, placebo-controlled, phase III trial evaluating primary efficacy and safety at twenty-four weeks. *Arthritis Rheum.* 2006;54(9):2793–2806.

36. Edwards JC, Szczepanski L, Szechinski J, et al. Efficacy of B-cell-targeted therapy with rituximab in patients with rheumatoid arthritis. *N Engl J Med.* 2004;350(25):2572–2581.

37. Kremer JM, Genant HK, Moreland LW, et al. Results of a two-year followup study of patients with rheumatoid arthritis who received a combination of abatacept and methotrexate. *Arthritis Rheum.* 2008;58(4):953–963.

38. Kremer JM, Genant HK, Moreland LW, et al. Effects of abatacept in patients with methotrexate-resistant active rheumatoid arthritis: a randomized trial. *Ann Intern Med.* 2006;144(12):865–876.

39. Kremer JM, Westhovens R, Leon M, et al. Treatment of rheumatoid arthritis by selective inhibition of T-cell activation with fusion protein CTLA4Ig. *N Engl J Med.* 2003;349(20):1907–1915.

40. Jones G, Sebba A, Gu J, et al. Comparison of tocilizumab monotherapy versus methotrexate monotherapy in patients with moderate to severe rheumatoid arthritis: the AMBITION study. *Ann Rheum Dis.* 2010;69(1):88–96. Epub.

41. Genovese MC, McKay JD, Nasonov EL, et al. Interleukin-6 receptor inhibition with tocilizumab reduces disease activity in rheumatoid arthritis with inadequate response to disease-modifying antirheumatic drugs: the tocilizumab in combination with traditional disease-modifying antirheumatic drug therapy study. *Arthritis Rheum.* 2008;58(10):2968–2980.

42. Emery P, Keystone E, Tony HP, et al. IL-6 receptor inhibition with tocilizumab improves treatment outcomes in patients with rheumatoid arthritis refractory to anti-tumour necrosis factor biologicals: results from a 24-week multicentre randomised placebo-controlled trial. *Ann Rheum Dis.* 2008;67(11):1516–1523.

43. Guidelines for monitoring drug therapy in rheumatoid arthritis. American College of Rheumatology Ad Hoc Committee on Clinical Guidelines. *Arthritis Rheum.* 1996;39(5):723–731.

F

Febuxostat, 157, 157*t*
Feet
 juvenile rheumatoid arthritis in, *36*
 pain in, 48, 49*t*, 55
 psoriatic arthritis in, *37*
 rheumatoid arthritis in, 85
Females
 anserine bursitis and, 54
 fibromyalgia and, 47
 giant cell arteritis and, 142
 idiopathic inflammatory myopathies and, 180
 relapsing polychondritis and, 190
 scleroderma and, 175
 Sjogren's syndrome and, 187
 systemic lupus erythematosus and, 109, 127
 Takayasu's arteritis and, 142
Fenofibrate, 158
Ferritin, inflammatory arthritis and, 90
Fibromyalgia, 6*t*, 15, 46, 46*t*, 57, 104–105
 features and prevalence of, 1*t*
 gender and, 47
 neck pain and, 69
Fingers, gout in, *42*
Finkelstein's test, 52
Flat foot, 48
Fluorodeoxyglucose PET, extracranial vasculitis and, 104
Fractures, osteoporosis and, 197
FRAX calculation, application of, 204
FRAX risk calculator, hip fracture in women and, 198–199*t*
Fungal arthritis, 5*t*
 diagnosis, 173
 laboratory studies, 172
 treatment, 173

G

Gastrointestinal disease, scleroderma and treatment for, 179*t*
Gastrointestinal tract, systemic lupus erythematosus and, 120
GCA. *See* Giant cell arteritis
Gender. *See also* Females; Males, Men; Women
 anserine bursitis and, 54
 fibromyalgia and, 47
 giant cell arteritis and, 101, 142
 idiopathic inflammatory myopathies and, 180
 low back pain and, 59
 osteoarthritis and, 71, 72*t*
 polymyalgia and, 101
 relapsing polychondritis and, 190
 rheumatoid arthritis and, 83, 84*t*
 scleroderma and, 175
 Sjogren's syndrome and, 187
 spondyloarthropathies and, 84*t*
 systemic lupus erythematosus and, 109, 127
 Takayasu's arteritis and, 142
General appearance, history, 14

Giant cell arteritis, 5*t*, 101, 137*t*, 142
 classification criteria for, 105*t*
 common clinical manifestations, 102–103
 common symptoms of polymyalgia rheumatica *vs.*, 103*t*
 diagnosis, 103–105
  differential, 104–105
  imaging, 103–104
  laboratory findings, 103
  tissue examination, 104
 epidemiology, 101
 ESR elevations in, 20
 features and prevalence of, 3*t*
 laboratory value changes associated with, 21*t*
 pathology/pathogenesis, 102
 treatment and clinical course of, 105–106
Glucocorticoid-induced osteoporosis, prevention and treatment of, 208–209*t*
Glucocorticosteroid therapy
 monitoring guidelines for rheumatoid arthritis, 219*t*
 systemic lupus erythematosus and, 124–125
Glucosamine chondroitin, osteoarthritis and, 75, 76
Gold, 95
"Golfer's elbow," 51
Golimumab, 96, 217
 dosing of, for rheumatoid arthritis, 218*t*
 monitoring guidelines for rheumatoid arthritis therapy, 219*t*
Gottron's rash, 11*t*, 181
Gout, 4, 5*t*, 11*t*, 151–158
 acute, 152
  colchicine and, 156
  corticosteroid joint injection for, 156
  IL-1 blocking agents and, 156
  joint immobilization and, 156
  management of, 155–156
  nonsteroidal anti-inflammatory drugs and, 155
  systemic corticosteroids and, 156
  workup of patient, 154–155
   history, 154
   imaging, 155
   joint aspiration, 154
   laboratory evaluation, 155
   physical examination, 154
 asymptomatic hyperuricemia, 151
 cause of, 151
 chronic tophaceous, 154
 clinical features and exam features/studies on, 8*t*
 features and prevalence of, 2*t*
 in fingers, *42*
 intercritical, 153
 uric acid-lowering therapies, 156–158, 157*t*
  recombinant uricases, 157*t*, 158
  uricosuric agents, 157–158, 157*t*
  xanthine oxidase inhibitors, 157, 157*t*
Gouty bursitis, 51
Guillain-Barre syndrome, 119
"Gull-wing" configuration, erosive osteoarthritis in hands and, *31*